permanent
waves

permanent
waves

The Making of the American Beauty Shop

Julie A. Willett

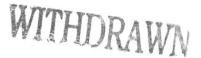
New York University Press   New York and London

New York University Press
New York and London

© 2000 by New York University

Library of Congress Cataloging-in-Publication Data
Willett, Julie A.
Permanent waves : the making of the American beauty shop /
Julie A. Willett.
p.   cm.
Includes bibliographical references and index.
ISBN 0-8147-9357-6 (cloth : alk. paper) —
ISBN 0-8147-9358-4 (paper : alk. paper)
1. Beauty shops—United States—History. 2. Beauty shopes—
Social aspects—United States.   I. Title.
TT957 .W54 2000
306.4—dc21   00-008394

New York University Press books are printed on acid-free paper,
and their binding materials are chosen for strength and durability.

Manufactured in the United States of America

10 9 8 7 6 5 4 3 2 1

For Dylan and Randy

Contents

Illustrations

Acknowledgments

This project began as a dissertation topic at the University of Missouri and owes much to the dynamic faculty and students I first met there. I want to thank especially Jean Allman, Maurice Manring, Mary Neth, Oleta Prinsloo, and Tom Sabatini, who all helped in tremendous ways. David Roediger inspired every page of this book as did Susan Porter Benson, whose friendship, advice, and scholarship I continue to cherish.

Many archivists, librarians, and friends also provided vital assistance during various stages of this project. The National Hairdressers and Cosmetologists Association, especially Robin Le Van of the Museum of Cosmetology, St. Louis, Missouri, graciously provided me access to the museum's collections. Vicky Jones of the Southwest Collection at Texas Tech University, Michael Flug of the Vivian G. Harsh Research Collection, Carter G. Woodson Regional Library, Ann Howe, Morris Fitch, Eric Bohle, and Terry Morris either were particularly helpful in finding photographs for this project or allowed me to use their own photographs, both contemporary and from years past.

In the final editing stages of this project Nancy Hewitt not only was encouraging but also provided a number of insightful suggestions. Kathy Peiss's comments and expertise in the study of beauty culture helped refine my own approach to the subject. Both Alywn Barr and Paul Deslandes also answered many questions on a range of subjects. I also want to thank my editor, Jennifer Hammer, who provided the comments I needed to pull it all together.

I owe much to my family who have helped me in many personal and professional ways. Lori Willett, while busy finishing her own doctorate, provided photos. Cindy Willett's research in social philosophy helped sort out various theoretical issues. My father, Joe Willett, kept me focused on the project, as did my mother, Ellen Willett, who also ran endless errands looking for anything from possible oral history interviews to contemporary articles about beauty shops and hair. Most important of all, Randy McBee along with our one-year-old son, Dylan, made this book not only possible but also a pleasure to write.

Acknowledgments

Introduction

My paternal grandmother lived most of her life in a small Missouri town located in the northwest corner of the state. As in many small towns, the beauty shop was central to the community and women's lives because it offered a place to socialize and pass the time as well as the chance to catch up on local gossip. The beauty shop that I recall my grandmother visiting was in the back of a barber shop. I remember on my occasional visit, walking through the barber shop with my grandmother in hand and being very conscious that we were somehow transgressing male space. The barber shop was not so different from my grandfather's harness repair shop in that it was filled with the same groups of men chewing tobacco and engaged in what seemed to me the same conversations about weather, politics, rodeos, and wrestling. Only the fixtures were different. The barber shop did not have a dirt floor or that pungent smell of leather, and a row of chairs stood in place of the more interesting display of western saddles.

Like these all-male hangouts in which my grandfather spent a good part of his time, the beauty shop was also a gender-specific place where my grandmother's work, leisure, and community life blurred together. My grandmother, along with many of her small-town friends, undoubtedly enjoyed their trips to the beauty shop, trips that were as much ritual as routine and often preceded special events that marked important moments in life. For my grandmother, social events, including everything from family reunions to visits from grandchildren, called for a special appointment and usually a new permanent. Indeed, besides the church, the beauty shop was the only place I ever remember my grandmother willingly leaving behind the comforts of her home or garden. And like my grandmother's church, the beauty shop was not so different from the porch culture where she, her sisters, and neighbors spent their leisure time and sorted out the politics of everyday life.[1] In the summers after dinner and dishes, my grandmother along with her close friends and relatives would sway back and forth on the porch swing, catching the occasional breeze, as they shared conversations, sometimes about gardening and canning and sometimes about more serious personal problems. Similarly, the beauty shop was a decidedly female space where a never-ending rumble of hair dryers and a multitude of conversations filled the air. For my grandmother and many of her friends and relatives, the church, the front porch, and the beauty shop were part of a larger women's culture that provided an invaluable source of information and the same types of social networks that historians have been so willing to see in saloons and other all-male institutions.[2]

Yet while the beauty shop was part of the community, it was also built on exclusion like the town of which it was a part. Just like many other small midwestern towns, my grandparents' hometown boasted a distinctively all-white population. Indeed, the town's collective memory recalls an all too familiar pledge that neither a "catholic or a nigger had ever spent the night in the town." As the town's folklore makes clear, its residents were certainly conscious of their whiteness, a consciousness that compelled them to boast about their racial and religious prejudice. My grandmother's beauty shop was also a reflection of the community it served. When my grandmother entered the beauty shop, she was not only entering a uniquely female sphere that allowed women to talk openly about the personal matters of home and family, but also a beauty shop that was as racially and ethnically exclusive as the town itself.

My grandmother's experience with beauty shops provides insight into the broader development of the industry in two distinct ways. First, like my grandmother, women have long embraced the beauty shop as an important part of a larger homosocial culture. Throughout the twentieth century, the beauty shop was first and foremost a place where women could enjoy the company of other women, and beauty shops remain places where women cherish female companionship, exchange information, share secrets, and either temporarily escape or collectively confront their problems and heartaches. Indeed, beauty workers would extend themselves personally and professionally to meet both the needs of their clients and the community, making the beauty shop, like the barber shop, an institution vital to culture, community formation, and social change.

At the turn of the century, there were only a few salons that catered to women and most of those were reserved for the more well-to-do. In the next two decades, however, changes in fashion and style, technological advances, and World War I compelled increasing numbers of women to search out their own beauty space. While operators who peddled their goods and services door-to-door met the beauty needs of some women, many others began patronizing local barber shops. Some barbers welcomed women into their shops and their increased profits. Others were much more ambivalent and feared that a woman's presence might disrupt or perhaps even eliminate the male culture to which barbers and their all-male clientele had grown accustomed. Just like saloons, barber shops played a crucial role in the public organization of masculinity throughout the early twentieth century.[3] The struggle over the nature of public space and the increasing desire among women to have their own homosocial space contributed to the dramatic growth of the women's hairdressing industry.

Second, the beauty shop was also a reflection of the racial segregation that has so profoundly shaped American society. According to African-American entrepreneur and activist Marjorie Stewart Joyner, there was a time before Jim Crow when whites and blacks frequented the same Chicago beauty shop. But, she continued, that was before segregation when blacks and whites still lived in the same neighborhood, an issue that has been ignored with regard to the beauty business.[4] In Lois Banner's cultural study of beauty and style in the late nineteenth and early twentieth centuries, she argues that women's participation in beauty rituals was central to women's separate culture and was linked to life experiences like childbirth and domestic work. But

4   of all the experiences to which historians have looked to define women's culture, Banner argues that "the pursuit of beauty, then as now, transcended class and racial barriers."[5] The beauty shop was indeed crucial to women's cultures, but these were cultures that also grew out of racial segregation and came of age with Jim Crow.

The history of women's hairdressing, then, is a history of two distinct industries which have different legacies yet share a similar past. Throughout most of twentieth century, the African American and Euro-American hairdressing industries traveled along divergent trajectories. From the standpoint of the white hairdressing industry, the black beauty shop was virtually invisible and financially insignificant until the 1970s. This invisibility along with the determination of black beauty operators to create their own employment opportunities allowed the African American hair-care industry to define itself on its own terms. From its origins to the present, the black-owned beauty shop consciously served both the needs of a female clientele as well as larger community and political goals. Thus its history, official and unofficial, recognized beauty workers as community leaders and beauty shops as important social institutions crucial to larger political struggles. In contrast, Euro-American hairdressing associations found themselves in a battle over self-definition that not only questioned the relationship between hairdresser and client, but also the sociability and the legitimacy of the small neighborhood shop.

Not all of the history of black and white hairdressers has been separate, however. While this study traces the development of two distinct industries, it also focuses on the points of intersection that correspond to key developments in the industry's history. African-American and Euro-American women faced similar work experiences that differed more by degree than by kind. Regardless of the shop in which they worked, women remained entrenched in a pink-collar ghetto where hazardous working conditions, low wages, long hours, and, most of all, a demanding and unpredictable clientele were common. By tracing the development of the hairdressing industry throughout the twentieth century, this study not only explores issues of work, skill, and professionalism unique to women's service work, but also how

African-American and Euro-American beauty workers responded
and attempted to carve out a work culture that met their own personal and professional needs.

The struggle to define beauty workers in terms of professionalism, especially within the context of the neighborhood shop, is crucial to understanding the industry's history and the degree to which it reflects the intersection of race, class, and gender. Although my grandmother's experience suggests that the beauty shop was inextricably bound to women's culture and community, the development of the Euro-American hairdressing industry reveals that this aspect of beauty shop culture was a point of contention. During the first half of the twentieth century, hairdressing associations such as the National Hairdressers and Cosmetologists Association (NHCA) defined themselves as the industry's leaders and concerned themselves primarily with regulating hairdressing and establishing it as a respected profession that fit neatly into the world of white-collar work and respectability. The NHCA, which was composed of exclusive shop owners, manufactures, and dealers, not only targeted wages and hours but also the small neighborhood shop that claimed ownership of a wide variety of home-grown beauty shop practices and products. Beauticians often mixed their own solutions and treated medical problems where they saw fit. Most important of all, the quest for professionalism signaled an attack on the female and working-class culture that had come to symbolize the small neighborhood shop, which made up the backbone of the industry. This struggle over professionalism reached its peak during the Depression when various trade associations and shop owners, through the establishment of National Recovery Administration (NRA) codes, attempted to set hours and wages that not only threatened the social organization of the hairdressing industry but also the existence of the popularly priced neighborhood shop. In short, the ethic of professionalism these industry leaders supported reflected their fear of being associated with women's work. Moreover, they were disproportionately white, middle-class, and male and tried to define the occupation in opposition to anything remotely feminine, domestic, and service-oriented. This meant ignoring the contributions of female hairdressers black or white and embracing an understanding of professionalism that defined

6   men as artists and women as mere gossip mongers and thus the bane of the hairdressing industry.

Ultimately, the professionalism the NHCA was trying to enforce was not only an attempt to disassociate the industry from women's work but also non-white service work. To a large degree, the quest for professionalism seemed a way to mollify the harsher side of the occupation—the long hours, the low pay, and the occupational hazards—but these were also characteristics that most blatantly contradicted its legitimacy and status as a respected white-collar occupation and were most readily associated with the female-dominated neighborhood shop. Above all, there was a conscious desire to rid the industry of workers whose very presence undermined this top-down definition of professionalism. In her study of nursing, Barbara Melosh found that the quest for professionalism meant "upgrading the workers," dismissing "'irregular' practitioners" and thus excluding "disproportionate numbers of socially marginal practitioners: black, immigrant, and white working-class men and women." Thus, Melosh argues that "professions are not just special organizations of work but rather particular expressions and vehicles of dominant class and culture."[6] Like the medical profession, Euro-American hairdressing associations worked to exclude anyone or anything that might undermine their sense of respectability and their definition of professionalism. In particular, this meant ignoring both the existence of the black hair-care industry and the history of the kitchen beautician whose home-grown hairstyling techniques, gossip, and cheap prices not only tainted the industry's reputation but placed it in an uncomfortably close association with non-white service occupations.

By the second half of the twentieth century, various trade associations and exclusive shop owners were still trying to enforce their own understanding of professionalism, but they along with various manufactures were also interested in expanding markets which ultimately meant restructuring the racial and gender boundaries that had long defined beauty shop culture. This desire for efficiency found its greatest support from the rise of more gender-neutral hairstyles and low-budget unisex chain salons, which were committed not only to bringing men and women into the same shop but also to rapid customer turnover. The corporate reorganization of the salon threatened the relationships upon which women had long based their identity and reflected a renewed interest and recognition of black consumers.

"Courting the ethnic market" quickly became the rallying cry for an industry that had for nearly two-thirds of a century been built on racial exclusion. As a result, white hairstylists increasingly reported being trained in black hair-care techniques, their trade journals began to include advertisements for black hair-care products, and black and white hairstylists were more likely to find themselves working shoulder to shoulder than during preceding decades. In short, the African-American beauty shop that had been ignored throughout the first half of the century had, by the 1970s, assumed an increasingly prominent position in the industry.[7]

The extent to which this group of industry leaders was successful in reorganizing the salon varied considerably. For most of the twentieth century, white hairstylists' understanding of skill, professionalism, and their very identity revolved around a racially exclusive shop. The introduction of chain salons and attempts to "court the ethnic market" threatened the boundaries around which beauty shops had developed as well as the hairstylist's position in the industry. To be more specific, corporate attempts to expand the industry disrupted the social organization of the beauty shop and challenged the intimacy that characterized relations between operator and customer, compelling both to resist industry changes. African-American hairdressers, for example, often sensed the white customer's discomfort, while white hairdressers increasingly articulated an unfamiliarity with "black hair" that questioned their own ability and skill to cut hair that they perceived as being so different from their own. Ultimately, then, the actions and attitudes of hairstylists and customers alike, who viewed the corporate reorganization of the industry as a threat to their identity, comfort, and sense of respectability, mitigated attempts to blur racial distinctions.

This study begins by examining the roots of the industry and capturing both its official and unofficial histories. In particular, the first chapter explores the ways in which gender, race, and class came to define the industry in the early twentieth century and how larger economic, cultural, and social changes shaped

8   women's work, consumer patterns, leisure habits, and sense of style. Such changes not only afforded women more money and opportunity, but also gave rise to new hair styles that had profound political ramifications for a generation of women coming of age during the first two decades of the twentieth century. These changes are woven through the official histories of the black and white hair-care industries, which have been constructed distinctly along lines of race. While African-American hair-care trade journals embraced the legacy of female entrepreneurs, the neighborhood shop, and political struggle, Euro-American hairdressing trade journals seemed to have little use for such stories and focused rigidly on technological progress and male ingenuity. Ultimately, the origins of the two industries reveal women's agency as workers and as consumers who were eager to define their own beauty space.

Chapter 2 examines the hopes, disillusionment, and resiliency of beauty workers as they struggled first to achieve entrance into the trade and then to create an acceptable work culture. More specifically, it looks at beauty school education, apprenticeship, and informal girlhood rituals of play and practice that provided entry into the trade. Operators faced diverse working conditions in the first third of the century. Because the industry was highly unregulated, beauty operators could be found in commercial establishments commonly located in department stores and business sectors but also in their homes, tenements, and even factory lavatories. Regardless of their surroundings, operators worked long and irregular hours, received low wages, and suffered injuries and health hazards, conditions which often became unbearable during the Depression. Because most shops were small and owner operated, workers' resistance was often individual and informal. Thus while some beauty operators sought collective organization, most turned to the rather precarious alliance they established with clients, whose loyalty was crucial in negotiating better wages and working conditions throughout the twentieth century.

Chapter 3 focuses more closely on the Depression and reform efforts designed to regulate an industry which had barely defined itself. Beauty operators who had just discovered the field of hairdressing confronted the hardships of the Depression while industry leaders attempted to limit the pool of operators and eliminate small competitors by setting up a rigid set of trade standards regulating everything from operating hours to prices. For the NHCA, the Depression exacerbated a crisis in professionalism that reflected the growing number of small-time beauty operators that worked in kitchens and front rooms rather than clearly defined business space. In a quest to save the profession from ruin, many hairdressing associations and shop owners demanded the regulation of the small neighborhood shop. The presence of the neighborhood shop with its distinctly working-class clientele, low prices, and late hours not only tainted the industry's reputation and legitimacy, but in the eyes of many was responsible for the trade's association with other non-white service work.

Chapters 4 and 5 look at changes and continuity in industry policies that had also characterized the first half of the twentieth century. In the face of World War II's labor shortages and postwar prosperity, the neighborhood shop became a useful example of how best to meet new consumer demands and community needs. Beauty shops were not only increasingly important to the everyday politics of women's lives but also to larger grassroots movements that challenged the system of apartheid upon which the industry and nation had been built. But whether or not beauty operators stepped out of their shops and into a larger community role, the beauty shop had become for many women regardless of race, class, or region a weekly routine. Almost overnight the causal atmosphere and the irregular hours that characterized the neighborhood shop and were once deemed unacceptable were hailed as the model for the industry as a whole. As well, the industry had learned an important lesson from the Depression— that flexibility was important to attract customers and sell hair products and services. No longer were white industry leaders interested in serving only the well-to-do. Bouffants and beehives along with the standing appointment meant a seemingly endless demand for beauty operators and supplies. Hailed as one of the fastest growing industries in the nation, the hairdressing industry now seemed to have room for both the upscale salon and the more modest neighborhood shop. Yet as the never-ending search for markets continued, race remained a rigid boundary.

Chapter 5 looks at the culmination of a century of struggle in which industry leaders and hairdressers, black and white, male and female, struggled with and against each other to establish the kind of salon that was profitable and best fit their own understanding of respectability. Cultural, social, and economic transformations since the 1960s ushered in new industry demands and the restructuring of the beauty shop that challenged the racial and gender boundaries that had long characterized hairdressing. More specifically, the growing popularity of carefree and low-maintenance hair styles and a desire for efficiency helped establish unisex chain salons that brought men and women into the same shop. At the same time, white corporate attempts to "court the ethnic market" threatened racial boundaries but did not undermine them as issues of race remained highly contested.

Throughout the twentieth century, the beauty shop has played an important role in women's lives. Not only has it remained a resource for female employment and entrepreneurship, but it has been crucial to culture and community. While bound to a much larger beauty industry, hairdressing has also emerged alongside other female-dominated service occupations such as retail sales and waitressing in which women as workers faced the contradictory demands of managers and customers. Thus the history of the beauty shop, like the department store and the restaurant, reveals the ways in which workers sought to negotiate decent wages, hours, and working conditions.[8] Throughout the first half of the twentieth century, women relied upon a number of different strategies to confront these workplace demands. By the second half of the century, women still confronted challenges to their work culture. But the racial segregation upon which the beauty industry had been founded was beginning to crumble. The expansion of the beauty industry, namely the rise of unisex chain salons and the attempts to attract black consumers, not only brought issues of gender into sharper relief but also those of race, challenging the exclusivity upon which the industry had been built and the manner in which generations of hairdressers had constructed their identity as workers and as professionals. Indeed, as with other industries, corporate America's attempts to more thoroughly dominate everyday life and restrict individual initiative led to intense struggles as workers and customers tried to create a salon similar to the small-town beauty shop in which my grandmother and her friends had come of age.

One final note to the reader: The sources I use reflect my determination to privilege the voices of the women who worked in the hairdressing industry. While trade journals, newspapers, and governmental investigations provide insight into industry-wide changes and corporate America's influence, I rely extensively on personal narratives, letters, and interviews that detail beauticians' day-to-day experiences. An extensive collection of Depression-era letters, for example, offers a rare glimpse into the lives of beauty workers as they coped with, manipulated, and resisted both the national cosmetology associations' efforts to dominate the industry and governmental attempts at regulation. Oral histories also reveal how beauticians fashioned their own identity and framed their resistance in an attempt to carve out autonomous spaces in this rapidly changing industry; such sources, however, are filled with the kind of inconsistencies in grammar and spelling that tend to characterize everyday speech and writing. To change such inconsistencies would undermine their richness and authenticity. Thus all quotes remain in their original form.

1

Getting to the Roots of the Industry

No one who has grown up in a multiracial society, however, is unaware of the fact that hair difference is what carries the real symbolic potency.

Orlando Patterson
Slavery and Social Death

In 1933, Gladys Porter began attending Douglas Junior High School in San Antonio, Texas, where she was "given a choice of vocational training in sewing, cooking, or beauty culture." Porter decided to pursue beauty culture and continued to take classes in high school. In order to become a certified beautician, she needed to complete a thousand hours of course work in a variety of subjects, including marcelling, permanent waving, croquignoling, shampooing, pressing, manicuring, scalp treatment, facials, and theory. Porter's all-black high school offered most of these courses, but it did not have a permanent-wave machine, a service offered almost exclusively in white-owned beauty shops. So she and her classmates made trips across town to a white high school where they received instructions on how to do permanent waves. Porter never forgot her visits to the white high school, especially the sense of discomfort she and her classmates felt each time they entered the classroom. In fact, she never exchanged a word with any of the white students—only the occasional glance, until one day outside of school, when she recognized a white student from her permanent-wave class. After a few awkward moments, Porter and her new friend began a "long conversation about the class" and quickly discovered that they shared a common concern— "the necessity of our having to learn to 'fix' the other race's hair."

Porter's new friend "could not understand why they wanted her to learn how to use a straightening comb and do colored folks' hair or why she should learn to use the steel curling iron." Porter agreed. "I couldn't understand why I should have to learn to do permanent waving and setting, adding that I had no desire to ever do white people's hair in the beauty shop that I hoped to open one day."[1]

The girls' attitudes were quite common. By the 1920s and 1930s, some white-owned beauty shops would hire African-American women to clean up the premises, shampoo a few heads, and occasionally even cut and style hair. But it was rare to find white women serving the beauty needs of African-American women. Trade journals reinforced the degree to which hairdressing emerged along distinct lines of race. Whether it was styles, tools, or techniques, the Euro-American hairdressing industry stood distinct from African-America beauty culture. But the differences do not stop there. Euro-American trade journals not only ignored the existence of the African-American hair-care industry, but also the contributions of female hairdressers regardless of race. While white, male hairdressers, who were cast as artists and entrepreneurs—beautifiers and businessmen—dominated the occupation's professional image, the history of the black hairdressing industry retold the stories of remarkable women such as Madam C. J. Walker, Annie Turnbo Malone, and Marjorie Stewart Joyner whose ideas and innovations transformed hairdressing into a respectable occupation and beauty shops into important community institutions.

This chapter explores both the hidden and the not so hidden roots of the hairdressing industry by documenting the pushes and pulls that first transformed kitchens and bathrooms into beauty parlors and turned domestic workers and farm girls into successful entrepreneurs. The histories of the African-American and Euro-American hairdressing industries' origins seem to differ more by degree than by kind. Looking at the cultural climate of the early twentieth century as well as the actions and attitudes of female workers and consumers, this chapter focuses on the connections between work and community as well as the relationship between politics and style, all of which made going to a beauty shop by the 1920s not simply a routine but a ritual that shaped and reshaped female identity throughout the life cycle. The integral connections between process and product, conversation and coiffeur, require a simultaneous examination of the beauty shop's work culture and the styles women wore in order to reveal how hair is "never a straightforward biological 'fact,'" but, in the words of Kobena Mercer, "a medium of 'significant' statements about self and society."[2]

The modern beauty shop owes much to African hairdressing traditions. In a biography of her great-great-grandmother Madam C. J. Walker, A'Lelia Perry Bundles emphasizes the connections between Walker's desire to create a career in beauty culture that served the needs of black women and her African heritage, connections that tell us much about hairdressing in the twentieth century.[3] In a study of African hairstyles, Esi Sagay defines hairdressing as an ancient art that dates as far back as the Egyptians and continues to be passed down from one generation of women to the next. "For the traditional hairdresser," Sagay finds, "hair is a medium for creative self-expression" that "requires artistry, manual dexterity and patience." African hairstyles and processes spoke not only to gender but also locality, lineage, and life cycle. The Fulani of West Africa, for example, styled children's hair in a fashion distinct from adults. Young girls would have their hair cornrowed or simply braided before marriage, while young boys would wear tufts of hair in various designs until circumcision, at which time their hair would be braided. As these young men matured, their plaits became more elaborate until they were married and their heads consequently shaven. Ceremonial occasions also called for intricate styles rich in tradition that, in turn, demanded skill and patience. Women spent hours, sometimes days, braiding and decorating hair. Many of these styles were so complex and demanded so much time to complete that a person might lay in the hairdresser's lap as their hair was arranged, an intimacy that would come to characterize the hairdresser-client relationship in America.[4]

In the United States, hairdressing not only remained an informal task rather than a clearly defined occupation, but also an important ritual that reaffirmed a sense of style and tradition. Under slavery, African Americans (while borrowing and blending European and Native American traditions) recreated hairstyling techniques that best suit the onerous tasks they performed day in and day out. With limited time and resources, many agricultural and domestic workers wore their hair quite short and used bandannas to protect their hair from the hot sun. The bandanna not only reduced the chance of heat stroke but, when wrapped tightly around the head, absorbed perspiration and "'trained' hair growth." Of course, wearing a "gaily-colored headkerchief" was never simply a matter of practicality. Not only did these "various colored turbans" articulate a cultural aesthetic that contrasted with the dominant European sense of color and pattern but the heat of the sun along with a bandanna could also be used to style hair. Former slaves remembered women wrapping or threading their hair with cotton and covering it with a bandanna in a manner Noliwe Rooks notes was not so different from the modern day practice of rolling hair on curlers and sitting under a dryer.[5]

Hair, however, took on its own unique and symbolic meaning within the larger confines of America's racial status quo, one that Orlando Patterson, in his comparative study of slavery, argues was more pervasive than skin color in establishing racial hierarchies. In the Americas, he contends, miscegenation quickly produced slave societies whose skin color was often lighter than the European masters. But hair, Patterson insists, was a different matter. "Differences between whites and blacks were sharper in this quality than in color and persisted for much longer with miscegenation," transforming hair into the "real symbolic badge of slavery." Patterson compares this phenomena to premodern societies where the shaving of a slave's head symbolized a loss of "manliness, power and 'freedom.'" Similarly, in modern societies, he argues, governments frequently shave the heads of prisoners to reinforce their subjugation. In the Americas, however, "blacks' hair was not shorn because, very much like the Ashanti situation where the slaves came with a readymade badge (their tribal tatoos), leaving the hair as it was served as a powerful badge of status," a distinction shaving would have undermined.[6]

Whether or not hair texture overshadowed skin color, the manner in which white settlers reacted to hair that did not fit neatly into their understanding of racial categorization further suggests its symbolic importance in defining America's racial hierarchies. If European hair was defined in terms of what it was not—e.g. "bushy," "kinky,"or "wooly"—then many slaves met their masters' and mistresses' own definition of beauty and refinement. Like the light-skinned slave who resembled his master a bit too much, long straight hair was a constant reminder that the racial ideologies upon which slavery was based were held together with the most transparent of contradictions. And when the hypocrisy became too much, it seems revengeful masters and mistresses lashed out with a vengeance. In Barbados in 1835, for example, the governor ordered that all slaves convicted of crimes have their hair shaven, something Patterson argues created a "golden opportunity" for mistresses who wished to put "'uppity' mixed female slaves in their place."[7] In the Antebellum South, former slaves also recalled that long hair, hair that was "fine as silk," often made the "Old Miss" envious and the mutilation of an African-American woman's hair a common form of punishment.[8] Similarly, in her mid-nineteenth century autobiography of life in the American South, Harriet Jacobs describes how her "fine head of hair" became the object of her master's fancy as well as his wrath. Indeed, Jacobs remembers that her master "often railed about my pride of arranging it nicely." But that was only when he thought he possessed her body, her beauty, and her pride. After Jacobs successfully undermined his sexual advances by orchestrating an affair with another man, her master became frustrated, "rushed from the house, and returned with a pair of shears." Jacobs never forgot how "He cut every hair close to my head, storming and swearing all the time."[9]

With the end of slavery, African-American women continued to struggle to assert their own sense of dignity, something they continued to do through style. After emancipation, freedwomen "carrying parasols and wearing veils" dismayed many white southerners. An officer of the Freedmen's Bureau reported that "the wearing of black veils by young negro women had given great offense to the young white women and that there was a time earlier in the season when the latter would not wear them at all."[10] As bell hooks explains, everywhere African-American women ventured in public, they were subjected to insults and "obscene comments" as well as physical assaults—all "at the hands of white men and women." In particular, an African-American woman who "dressed tidy and clean" or carried "herself in a dignified manner, was usually the object of mud-slinging by white men who ridiculed and mocked her self-improvement efforts."[11]

White vengeance, however, merely made African-American women more determined to look, dress, and act the way they wanted. Indeed, beauty culture was in many ways a world-wide reaction to the problems African descendants faced as well as the Eurocentric notions of beauty and refinement they encountered. Whether it was music, dance, cookery, or dress, Kobena Mercer points out, "black peoples of the African Diaspora have developed distinct, if not unique, patterns of style" in response to the common "experience of oppression and dispossession." In particular, Mercer writes, hair-styling became a means to articulate "a variety of aesthetic 'solutions' to a range of 'problems' created by ideologies of race and racism."[12]

Hairdressing in the United States also reinforced racial hierarchies as it became yet another service in which black labor catered to white needs. Through the nineteenth century a small minority of free African-American women worked as hairdressers in northern towns and cities, but they generally catered to white upper-class women rather than African Americans. As Eliza Potter describes in her 1859 autobiography, hairdressing afforded her an unusual degree of independence and privilege. Yet the occupation was one she ultimately characterized as problematic. While the skills of a good hairdresser were highly valued, she also implied that the black hairdresser was treated just like the domestic servant, privy to the personal lives of the women to whom they catered, even fulfilling the role as confidant, yet ultimately dismissed as an outsider whose presence and labor existed simply to cater to white vanity.[13] Similarly, in the slave South, African Americans often took care of their masters and mistresses' personal needs, including styling and washing their hair. Elizabeth Fox-Genovese argues that house servants "took pride in having their mistress always look their best and outshine the other ladies."[14] But this was not the kind of satisfaction that would galvanize the development of an entire industry. In fact, in the 1890s, W. E. B. Du Bois found that barbering in Philadelphia, which had "for so long" been considered "almost exclusively [a]

Negro calling," had fallen out of favor because African-American barbers were increasingly forced to draw a color line and cater only to white men, something Du Bois thought "smacks perhaps a little too much of domestic service," while ultimately redefining barbering as "a thing to fall back upon but not to aspire to."[15]

By the early twentieth century, an African-American hairdressing industry that served black clients was becoming more visible, but many of these hairdressers were still relying on white consumer dollars to make ends meet. In 1896, Mrs. Grace Garnett-Abeny operated a beauty parlor at 2808 South State Street in Chicago, "just across from Emmanuel Jackson's undertaking business." Although she established the business especially for African Americans, Abeny catered to both black and white women. According to Abeny, her clientele came primarily from Chicago's "upper class Negroes," who she noted were of "mixed blood."[16] A decade later, Chicago beautician and soon-to-become political activist, Marjorie Stewart Joyner was accepted to an all-white beauty school but was also trained to do African-American styles. She opened a beauty shop at 54th and 48th Streets and "did a landslide business because it was one of the first shops for white and black." In those days, Joyner recalled, "you see black and white used to live together."[17]

While the few beauty shops that existed in the early 1900s may have catered to both African-American and Euro-American customers, less than a generation later the institution had undergone dramatic change and had become as rigidly segregated as the neighborhoods and communities to which it was intimately linked. In 1935, the Women's Bureau found few African-American women styling white women's hair and there were no cases provided in any investigations of white hairdressers with a steady black clientele.[18] Indeed, by the 1930s, the Chicago hairdressing industry had become rigidly divided along lines of race. In their study of Chicago's "black metropolis," St. Clair Drake and Horace R. Cayton found no white-owned or operated beauty parlors or barber shops in Chicago's black neighborhoods. "If colored undertakers have virtual monopoly in burying the Negro dead," then Drake and Cayton concluded, "the colored barber and beautician have even more exclusive monopoly in beautifying the living."[19]

The hairdressing industry's racial segregation may have reflected the refusal of whites to serve the needs of black customers or their reluctance to venture into predominantly black neighborhoods. But it also reaffirmed hairdressing as a means to carve out some space free from white oppression and reflected African-American desires for economic independence. Lizabeth Cohen, for example, found that during the 1920s, "a consensus developed in the black community that a separate 'black economy' could provide the necessary glue to hold what was a new and fragile world together." If African-American consumption could support a separate economy, this in turn would create jobs as well as businesses and institutions specifically designed to benefit African Americans.[20] As workers, consumers, and community members, African-American women sought to turn beauty culture into an industry that catered exclusively to black needs. More specifically, countless numbers of domestic workers chose hairdressing as a means to escape white kitchens, white households, and white control.

According to Marjorie Stewart Joyner, "In those days, back in 1915, . . . you had to create a job in order to have a job."[21] And create they did. At the turn of the century, the black hairdressing industry began as a door-to-door cottage industry. By 1916, Madam Walker alone employed 20,000 agents. While most of her employees were located in the United States, she also expanded her business to Central America and the Caribbean.[22] At the turn of the century, Annie Turnbo Malone was manufacturing Wonderful Hair Grower and finding financial success "canvassing house to house, [and] treating hundreds of scalps personally." By the 1920s, she had more than 60,000 representatives.[23] Unlike the Euro-American side of the industry, which originated as strictly service work, many African Americans also peddled hair and beauty products door-to-door. Nevertheless, the number of beauty shops catering to an exclusively black clientele also increased rapidly throughout the country. In 1920, the U.S. census found that 12,660 African-American women were working as "female barbers and hairdressers."[24] And by the 1930s, the president of the National Beauty Culturists Association, Rosilyn Stewart, reported that African-American beauty shops employed 150,000 women and were located in seventy-two cities and thirty-four states. Beauty shops could be found in the West, Midwest and South, but the majority were in the Northeast, particularly in places like New York City. In New York, the State Department of Labor found that in general African-American women "spoke enthusiastically of beauty parlor work as a new opening for Negro women and a field which offers opportunities for better wages and more independence than most work available for them."[25]

The growth and popularity of the beauty industry in part reflected the lack of alternatives open to black women. Jacqueline Jones argues that by World War I, northern black female wage work was "synonymous with domestic service." In cities such as New York and Chicago, African-American women made up one-fifth of all domestic workers. In Philadelphia, the percentage of black women who worked as domestics was over half, and in Pittsburgh, over 90 percent of the black female population was employed as day workers, washerwomen, or live-in servants.[26] While increased employment opportunities may have attracted black migrants to the urban north, few newcomers were able to find work in businesses that African Americans owned and operated. Instead, female migrants found themselves in urban centers where racial segregation along with class and gender restrictions limited the types of jobs available, leading an overwhelming number of African-American women to become household workers.[27] Madam C. J. Walker, for example, had been a laundress before opening up her own business.[28] And her successor, Marjorie Stewart Joyner, was doing "house work after school" when a friend asked, "why don't you get some regular work something you can depend upon." Hairdressing, her friend pointed out, would allow a woman to own her own business. And as her friend explained, with hairdressing, "you will always have a job" and "something to do because there is always somebody that wants their hair fixed on account of personal appearance."[29] Another Walker agent, Lizzie Bryant, perhaps best captures the benefits of hairdressing. "I have all I can do at home," boasted Bryant, "and don't have to go out and work for white people in kitchens and factories."[30]

African-American women did find some work beyond the confines of white households, but the alternatives available in industry also brought little satisfaction. Instead, many industrial jobs

were made available simply because white women rejected them.
Like African-American men, black women worked primarily in
physically demanding, dirty, and dangerous workplaces. Black
women worked in glass and tobacco factories, butchering and
meat processing, and sea food industries, under what they aptly
described as "disgusting conditions." In 1930, one quarter of all
African-American wage earners worked in poorly ventilated, unbearably hot and humid commercial laundries. Yet even these jobs
were scarce. In 1910, only 3 percent of African-American women
working for wages had jobs in manufacturing. And by 1930, the
figure had only risen to 8 percent. During and after World War I,
black women continued to be denied access to "good jobs" with
better wages and more tolerable working conditions. In addition,
white women were also known to refuse to work or eat with black
women and even demanded separate rest rooms and cafeterias,
something few employers were willing or able to afford. When
Euro-American businesses hired black women, store owners
often complained that they lost customers because the general
public refused to interact with African-American saleswomen or
secretaries. Even in predominantly black neighborhoods, white-
owned businesses refused to hire African Americans "for anything but menial jobs." For example, while clerical and sales jobs
accounted for one-third of all white women's employment in
1930, the same occupations accounted for only 1 percent of
African-American women's paid labor. As white women left domestic service and moved into more prestigious occupations, the
percentage of African-American household laborers continued to
rise, reaching 54 percent in 1930.[31] It was within this context that
Lizzie Bryant so nicely juxtaposed the advantages of beauty culture with the limitations of household labor and factory work.[32]

Beauty culture also allowed black women the chance to escape
the horrendous problems associated with white households. On
the one hand, domestic work severely limited the time they could
spend caring for their own families, something which was especially problematic if they were "live-in" rather than household
day workers. As Elizabeth Clark-Lewis argues, live-in employment forced women to not only live in small cramped quarters, but such work also isolated them from their communities. In
her study of Washington, D.C., Lewis found that one of the most

common complaints resulted from the inability to regularly attend Sunday services, which for some women came to symbolize the gravest restrictions of live-in household labor.[33] On the other hand, African-American women who worked in white households were more likely to suffer from sexual exploitation at the hands of white men. "I believe nearly all white men take, and expect to take undue liberties with their colored female servants—[and] not only the father, but in many cases the sons also," stated one household worker. Nor was it a situation easily resolved. "Those servants who rebel against such familiarity must either leave or expect a mighty hard time, if they stay."[34] Looking back at her childhood, civil-rights activist Bernice Robinson chose a career in beauty culture because of similar concerns. Robinson's mother insisted that none of her daughters work in white homes. "I don't ever want any girl of mine to do any domestic work or work in these white folks' kitchens." Robinson "understood" exactly "what was on her [mother's] mind." "If you do domestic work," she made clear, "and the white man comes home and he wants to have sex with you, you can't do anything about it. You have to give in." And Robinson's mother "wasn't going to have that with her girls."[35]

It is not surprising, then, that the founders of the industry often understood beauty culture as crucial to the all-around success of African-American women—socially, economically, politically, and even spiritually. Linked to race progress, good grooming, education, thriftiness, and hard work were all elements of the "politics of respectability," and one of the many ways African-American men and women tried to undermine notions of white supremacy. "Respectability," Evelyn Brooks Higginbotham argues, "was perceived as a weapon . . . used to expose race relations as socially constructed rather than derived by evolutionary law or divine judgement."[36] For example, Annie Turnbo Malone, whose products by the 1940s included everything from hair grower, pressing oil, and tetter salve to lipstick, rouge, and face powder and sold throughout the country, believed that beauty culture was a means of self-realization and important to a broader self-help ideology.[37] In a fashion similar to that of missionaries, Malone began in Missouri and then traveled to nearby states, "lecturing in churches, talking to groups, anywhere, everywhere,

the burden of her plea being the hygienic importance of a clean
scalp and the value of beautiful hair." Malone proclaimed "that
clean scalps encouraged clean bodies, that better appearance
meant greater business opportunities, higher social standing,
cleaner living and beautiful homes." According to a biographer,
Poro College, Malone's St. Louis-based training facility, was never
simply about dressing hair. Rather, her students were "her disci-
ples and agents [who] broadcast the message, and spread what became almost a racial culture."[38] Poro College, for example, was described as a "place where training does not confine itself to the
handling of hairdressers tools, but embraces all that the word
'beauty' implies—beauty of thought, of spirit; the beauty of
cleanliness, of grace, of dignity, of Godliness: the beauty of service and above all, the beauty of living." Thus Malone understood
beauty culture not merely as a trade or a field of study, but rather
a solution to society's ills. "First in its field," Poro brought in "the
realization to a whole race of people that appearance is the magic
'open sesame' to the many opportunities that otherwise would be
denied us." Ultimately, Malone's "fondest hope" was that soon
men, too, will "come into the same consciousness of the value of
proper grooming as have the women of the race."[39]

As Malone's biographer suggests, then, beauty culture developed hand-in-hand with notions of race progress. But like the
broader movement of which it was a part, hairdressing was also
embroiled in controversy. Throughout the early twentieth century, the mass marketing of hair products and skin creams that
promised to straighten hair and lighten skin tainted the entire industry. Products with names like "Black-No-More and Tan Off,"
Kathy Peiss argues in her study of the cosmetic industry, "baldly
appealed to European aesthetic standards and the belief that
light-skinned African Americans were more successful and, if
women more desirable as wives."[40] Indeed, Madam Walker, who
was credited with inventing the "straightening comb," was frequently accused of advocating similar aesthetic standards, although black leaders were reluctant to be too critical. Caught between products and producers whose messages seemed self-
loathing yet whose profits were undeniable, men like Marcus
Garvey denounced bleaching and straightening yet advertized
whitening creams and pressing oil in his paper the *Negro World*.[41]

In response, Madam Walker often diffused criticisms of her beauty culture products by creating what Noliwe Rooks characterizes as a "loud silence in her advertisements," which meant asking editors and writers to refrain from using the term "hair straightener" within a newspaper or magazine's text. Above all, she asserted that "the ritual of her system was as important as the actual hairstyle." Walker instructed her agents to create a safe and comfortable place in which African-American women could, for a change, be the ones who were pampered.[42] Walker believed this kind of personal attention and pampering gave black women the self-confidence to endure the harsher reality of their lives. In particular, Walker agents learned from her textbook that beauty "does not refer alone to the arrangement of the hair, the perfection of the complexion or to the beauty of the form. . . . To be beautiful, one must combine these qualities with a beautiful mind and soul."[43]

Madam Walker also challenged her critics by ensuring that her business remain committed to the community, something that in turn further enhanced the profession's status. Not only were African-American beauty operators relatively free from white control, but they also had the means to give back to the community. Whether it was black schools, orphanages, or civil rights organizations, Walker contributed generously while immersing herself in political struggles such as the rights of black World War I veterans and the fight for federal antilynching legislation. After the St. Louis Race Riot of 1917, she along with "a number of Walker agents" helped galvanize some 10,000 black New Yorkers in the Negro Silent Protest Parade that July. Walker, in collaboration with other black leaders, including James Weldon Johnson and W. E. B. Du Bois, also petitioned the White House, demanding "that lynching and mob violence be made a national crime punishable by the laws of the United States." In her struggle for civil rights, she maintained that all of her beauty-culture agents "become community leaders [and] political lobbyists."[44] With this, the beauty shop had clearly defined its position as a political outpost within black communities.

Although Madam Walker died in 1919, she established an important precedent for her contemporaries as well as future generations. Her mentor and contemporary, Annie Turnbo Malone,

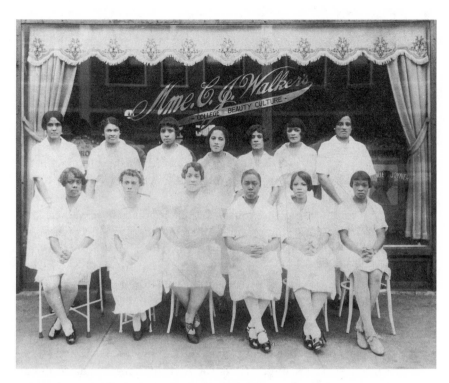

First graduates, Madame C. J. Walker College of Beauty Culture, 1926. Courtesy of Vivian G. Harsh, Collection of Afro-American History and Literature, Carter G. Woodson Regional Library, Chicago, Ill., Marjorie Stewart Joyner Collection.

continued to contribute generously to black organizations: thousands of dollars went to the Pine Street Y.M.C.A., to Howard University's Medical Endowment Fund, to the City-Wide Y.M.C.A. Campaign of St. Louis, and to St. Louis' Orphan's Home, and there were countless gifts to black schools, churches, and other institutions. In times of extreme need, Malone provided her community with relief. For example, after a tornado devastated St. Louis in 1927, Malone was "one of the principal relief units of the American Red Cross." In fact, "thousands of storm sufferers were sheltered, clothed and fed thru Poro College."[45] Similarly, Madam Sara S. Washington, founder of Apex News and Hair Company, began her business in 1918 on a "shoestring" in Atlantic City. Through hard work, she, like her predecessors, managed to build a successful manufacturing business from modest means, eventually producing seventy-five different Apex products while employing over two hundred workers and more than thirty-five thousand Apex agents "throughout the world." Her success allowed her to give financial support back to her community. Most notably, she renovated a "Home for Girls" in Atlantic City, which was used as a recreation center, and she contributed to The Home for Afflicted Children. During times of crisis, such as the "severe winter months" of the Great Depression, Washington, with the help of local civic organizations, gave away tons of coal to the city's poor.[46]

By contributing generously to their communities, Walker, Malone, and Washington served as formidable role models whose actions and attitudes attracted women to the field of beauty culture and helped legitimize an industry that was under close scrutiny. Above all, they were instrumental in creating a definition of professionalism that was community based and would in years to come challenge top-down notions of professionalism that ignored women's work and cultures. While the degree of their success was unique, their achievements, community involvement, and political activism were indicative of the African-American hairdressing industry throughout the twentieth century. Beauty shops were one of the few independently-owned businesses. They provided women a safe space away from obtrusive employers and white households which, in turn, allowed African-American women to construct community institutions and positions of leadership that would play an important role in black communities and shape the industry for years to come.[47]

Similar to African-American hair-care practices, Euro-American women throughout the nineteenth century rarely had their hair professionally washed and styled. The NHCA found that prior to World War I, "the services of cosmetologists were restricted to the 'privileged classes,' 'women of theatre,'" and those who "had the courage to brave the social-moral stigma that attached itself then to 'artificial embellishment.'"[48] In fact, throughout the late nineteenth century it took a city of 70,000 inhabitants to support one business.[49] As a result, hair care was an informal do-it-yourself task that only gradually transformed into a thriving service industry in the 1920s. Whether it was collecting rain water to rinse hair, making shampoo, or grooming children's hair, mothers and daughters not only shared in the activity at hand but passed the tradition of caring for hair and scalp down from one generation of women to the next. And even when a special occasion demanded a more elaborate do, women simply used old rags, pieces of cloth, or old chicken bones to set the hair overnight and temporarily transform straight hair into curly locks.[50]

During this same time, the men and women who considered themselves "ladies' hairdressers" generally spent their time and earned their money washing, combing, and arranging hair rather than cutting it. Ida Connolly, who began working as a "beauty operator" in Rochester, Minnesota in the 1910s, recalled that the beauty shop was as much about cleanliness as style. When Connolly first began working as a hairdresser, she found that the length of hair made the job itself a somewhat tedious process that tested the patience of hairdresser and customer alike, for considerable time and skill were needed simply to get the "snarls out of some long dragging lock." It seemed "Everyone had long hair" back then, Connolly recalled, "and it took half a day to take care of each client," something that effectively limited the beauty clientele to those with a certain degree of free time and money.[51] Adele Leffert of St. Joseph, Missouri, also recalled women's long hair. According to her mother, who was living in Cripple Creek, Colorado, in the late 1890s, "Back then women and girls had long hair and usually wore it in braids or in a bun at the back of the head," or a curling iron, which was heated by sticking it "down in the glass chimney of an oil lamp," was used to "curl the hair around the face."[52]

Immigration only seemed to reinforce the tradition of long hair and the limited role of the hairdresser. Through the first couple decades of the twentieth century, most southern and eastern European immigrant women rarely cut their hair. Elizabeth Ewen notes that in Italy the hairdresser might visit a woman's home on occasion. "Since water was scarce," Ewen found that "hair was not washed frequently; instead for a few cents a month the hairdresser came to the house to arrange, brush, and oil the women's hair." In America, the hairdresser served a similar purpose.[53] Rose Tellerino, who immigrated to the United States in 1900 and married in 1913 at the age of fourteen, noted that she became a mother

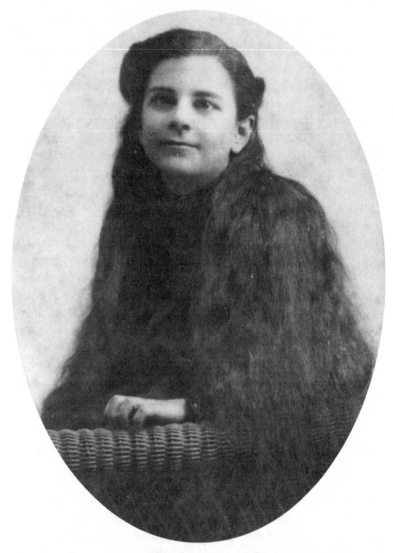

Angie Bryan Johnson before the "bob," c. 1912. From the author's collection.

in 1916. By seventeen, she complained that she probably looked thirty-seven, in part, because of the rigors of marrying so young and having a child. But also, she claimed, because of her long hair. "It ain't like today" when "they cut hair," she stated, suggesting that at least through the first two decades of the twentieth century most women simply had their hair washed or combed out instead of cut.[54]

On the eve of World War I, "everyone still considered it [hairdressing] to be only a fad." Unlike Marjorie Stewart Joyner, whose family and friends encouraged her to take up hairdressing, Connolly found that few friends or family members considered it a legitimate occupation, suggesting that the black hairdressing industry had not only matured somewhat earlier but that the development of beauty shops was uneven, gaining popularity first in large urban areas, then in smaller towns and farming communities. And even when some of these shops opened their doors, many seemed skeptical that the beauty shop would ever become a permanent institution. Connolly, for example, was warned that the "ladies would return to the old ways of shampooing and dressing their hair themselves." Connolly's mother in particular was "disgusted" at the thought of her daughter giving up a decent job in a hotel that paid eight dollars a week to simply "wash hair" and quite certain that "nobody was going to spend money

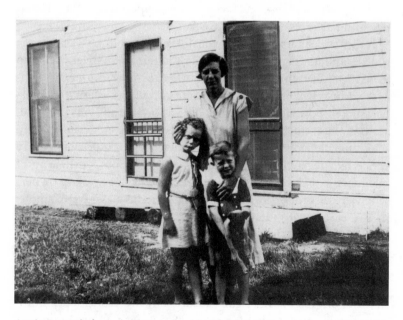

Angie Bryan (Johnson) McCown "bobbed" with children in front of her mid-Missouri home during the Depression. From the author's collection.

Getting to the Roots of the Industry

to have their hair fixed in a beauty parlor." If they did, her mother maintained, "It was just a momentary fad!," convincing Connolly that her mother might be right.[55]

Beauty shops, of course, became much more than just a "fad." Between 1910 and 1920 the number of "female barbers and hairdressers" increased by more than 10,000 raising the number of women in hairdressing to just over thirty-three thousand.[56] The number of shops grew at an equally dramatic pace. In 1920, there was a mere 5,000 shops in the United States. By the end of the decade, that figure had increased to 40,000 shops nationwide.[57] While this estimate included all kinds of shops, it undoubtedly overlooked the hundreds if not thousands of businesses tucked away in kitchens and tenement flats known only by word of mouth and operating in the most informal of fashions. In fact, what Connolly feared was a fad on the eve of World War I was quickly becoming a working girls' routine. At Mrs. Smith's beauty shop where Connolly worked, the clientele not only included the banker's wife but also store clerks and school teachers. And even Connolly's friend Kathleen, whom she described as a "simple little waitress, made a standing appointment for a shampoo and hair dress every two weeks."[58]

Industry leaders generally considered the industry's dramatic growth and its origins to be the result of European inventions and male ingenuity. In contrast to the African-American beauty-culture industry, Euro-American trade associations ignored hairdressing's more feminine and homegrown traditions and described the industry's origins in terms of male achievement and scientific development, and not women's work or community concerns. In particular, the NHCA was composed primarily of manufactures, dealers, school owners, and exclusive shop owners who were disproportionately male and middle-class. For example, in the early 1930s, Emile Beauvais, who was president of the NHCA, owned a "fine establishment" in Washington, D.C. that not only offered "four floors dedicated to the grooming and beautification of women," but was best known in "social, diplomatic, and political circles."[59] Not surprisingly, Beauvais understood that the origins of American hairdressing were decidedly European, male, and technological. "The Beauty Shop industry," Beauvais claimed, was a "very old one . . . brought to this coun-

try from Europe before the founding of the Republic." Only "a
generation ago," he asserted, hairdressers were men, "but it is
now and has been for many years conceded to be essentially a
woman's business," offering women one of the few opportunities
to own their own businesses. The feminization of the industry, he
continued, occurred because of "two things": the "Bob," a short
hairstyle, which "forced women . . . to seek the services of a hairdresser or barber, and the invention of the permanent wave."
The impact of these two developments was so "great," he declared, that existing businesses simply failed to meet the new
demand.[60]

The NHCA's official history agreed with Beauvais, emphasizing
key changes in style and European experiment and innovation.
On the one hand, the NHCA stressed that the expansion of the industry reflected the practical choices and problems women confronted. The U.S. entrance into World War I, for example, opened
new positions for women who found themselves at the front
working as nurses, stretcher-bearers, ambulance-drivers, or at
home working in ammunition plants and as factory hands—occupations traditionally filled by men and "regarded as impossible
for women." At the front, women soon found that they had little
time to care for their appearances. Short hair was easier to keep
clean than long hair and provided the best "defense against ver-
min." Moreover, female ammunition factory workers found that
long hair and gun powder were a dangerous combination.
Wartime newspapers, which filled their pages with "photographs
of women wearing overalls, knickers, and with hair bobbed,"
only enhanced the popularity of the style. Other women, "learning of the comfort and time-saving qualities of short hair, soon
took up the practice." By the end of the war, so the story goes, the
bob showed some signs of fading out, but was revived by mov-
ing-picture actresses, especially Irene Castle, "of the famous
dance team."[61]

On the other hand, the NHCA highlighted the contributions of
certain men. In particular, the NHCA cited the work of Parisian
Marcel Grateau, who in 1872 after several attempts with a curling
iron "to complete a broken natural wave in his mother's hair, by
accident reversed the iron and formed a flat wave." Three years
later he achieved what came to be "known as a 'marcel wave' on

straight hair," a style that would remain popular through the 1930s and '40s. In 1879, another French hairdresser, Alexandre F. Godefroy, who a contemporary described as the "king of hairdressers," was credited with the invention of the hot-blast hair dryer, which dramatically increased the number of women patronizing the "hairdressing parlor" as "milady could have her long tresses shampooed and dried in an hour instead of the drying process requiring almost an entire day by the palm leaf fan method." Last but not least, Charles Nessler, a German hairdresser, was hailed not only as the inventor of the permanent-wave machine, but according to *Time* magazine a "revolutionist," who "transformed women's way of life." Such "time-saving inventions," namely the permanent-wave machine and the hair dryer, made trips to the beauty shop more convenient for "working women." Hence, the NHCA, an organization that these men helped establish, continued to focus on these turn-of-the-century inventions, inventions many claimed "revolutionized the grooming habits of women throughout the world."[62]

While the NHCA credited these men with the inventions that ushered in a new industry and trade journals spent a considerable amount of time and money advertising new styles and techniques, their influences on beauty-shop practices were ambiguous at best. Some women simply ignored trade publications and advice. Ida Connolly recalled being bombarded with the new innovations of the 1920s. And although she "would read different articles on the subject," she admitted that she "kept right at work in the same old ways," as if many beauty operators preferred to stay with the methods they and their customers were most comfortable with rather than follow trade-journal advice. Female beauty workers also jerry rigged their own inventions. Connolly, for example, first used a hair dryer—but it was not Godefroy's invention but rather a "rigged up" hair dryer invented by her employer, Mrs. Smith. "It was simply a chair placed in front of the gas stove, with a horn similar to that of an old Victrola, made at the black-smith's shop, with a fan in back of the stove, to direct the hot air onto the head." It was slow and cumbersome, Connolly recalled, but it worked.[63] Nor was the permanent-wave machine strictly a European original. African-American entrepreneur Marjorie Stewart Joyner invented a permanent-wave machine

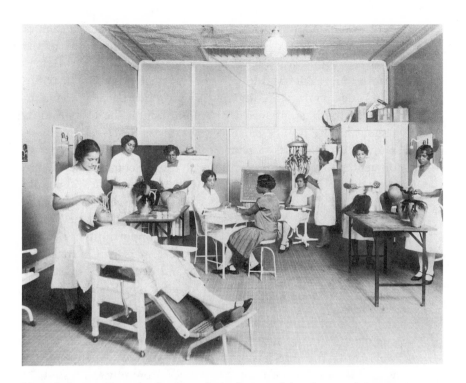

Marjorie Stewart Joyner's salon in 1928. At the rear of the photograph Joyner is seen working on a customer with her patented permanent-wave machine. Courtesy of Vivian G. Harsh, Collection of Afro-American History and Literature, Carter G. Woodson Regional Library, Chicago, Ill., Marjorie Stewart Joyner Collection.

and, although her version was never marketed, she held "all the patents and everything." With the help of her nephew and a cousin, Joyner described how they "made up two or three as best we could and I used them until I got more involved in the schooling aspect of this business, teaching rather than staying in the shop." Joyner knew the ins and outs of the industry and was well aware that "nobody in the business at the time wanted anything that would take away their method and push mine." And since she "didn't have the money," she never marketed her invention. "Mine was faster," she asserted, "but since it belonged to me, they didn't want it" and hence it remained hidden from the NHCA's official history.[64]

Female ingenuity also accounts for the dramatic expansion of the beauty industry. As Kathy Peiss finds in her study of the cosmetics industry, women such as Elizabeth Arden and Helena Rubinstein "redefined and pioneered techniques in distribution, sales, and marketing that would later become commonplace in the businessworld."[65] And although she was never as famous as the beauty culturists that Peiss describes, Ida Connolly and thousands of women like her encouraged the development of beauty culture often relying on common sense and their own brand of business savvy. In many cases, it was simply a matter of being available regardless of time or place. In the early years when women first began to have their hair professionally styled, Connolly never let any opportunities slip by. On a somewhat regular basis, her customers would make up their minds at the very last minute and decide they must have their hair cut that evening, hours after the beauty shop on Broadway had closed. Fearful they might change their mind, Connolly put aside whatever she was doing to please a potential customer. "I might just be home after my day's work on Broadway, my own dinner preparations just started" when someone would knock on the door. Sometimes, Connolly confessed, "I had to turn that [house]work over to our dear Grandma and get out the shears and a towel to please some customer who had followed me home." Doing hair after hours was never a trade-journal suggestion, nor did the NHCA ever advice beauty operators to carry their scissors and combs with them just in case unexpected customers made an appearance. Yet by doing just that, Connolly successfully courted her clientele. Even on Sunday at a church picnic "two ladies, then three, clustered about me in a great conference," all demanding their hair be bobbed. When it was finally time "for eats," Connolly found "the picnic ground covered with hair and a critical audience of most of the ladies waiting their turn." "What a busy person I was then," Connolly recalled no doubt reflecting upon her unconventional yet undeniable entrepreneurial success.[66]

Beauty operators also understood that bobbing hair was not a simple decision for many women. Connolly remembered when the "new fad had hit the hair-conscious ladies," everyone started to think about the implications of such a dramatic change in feminine style. Customers would stop by, Connolly explained, but they were usually hesitant and often in need of some coaxing. The first to try the new look were always "the more daring." But even these customers would insist that she go slow and not cut off "too much at first." Sometimes the process was long and drawn out for customers "would dare to have only half of their hair cut, either the front or the back." At times, they would flee the shop in tears regretting what they had done. But, with a little persuasion and a lot of patience, "it wouldn't be too long before they would be back to have the rest cut off," transforming what had once been a daring adventure into a regular routine.[67]

Female beauty operators also offered their customers personal experience as expertise, something that put male hairdressers and manufactures at a distinct disadvantage. When Charles Nessler began to market his permanent-wave machine, he found that women were often afraid of such a strange looking contraption, compelling him to tour the country and put on a series of free demonstrations for old and young alike.[68] But it took more than a few celebratory demonstrations to make the permanent wave a beauty shop ritual. Indeed, it was only after beauty operators themselves became comfortable using the apparatus that it caught on and even then Connolly's customers questioned its reliability: "Will it really stay?" Connolly was repeatedly asked as she patiently explained the process of having a permanent wave, reassuring each new customer that "It is really possible to take perfectly straight hair and within three hours make it stay curled until it grows out." When words failed to convince her skeptical clients, Connolly dabbled in self experimentation and made a trip "to the Twin Cities with four other girls who were going up" to try out the new invention. Connolly's hair was "just as fuzzy as it could be," and much to her customers' disbelief "it didn't wash out," proving that the beauty operators' ability to share their female client's "bodily trials and tribulations" was one of the best tricks of the trade.[69]

The hairdressing industry also grew dramatically because it offered Euro-American women a certain amount of satisfaction missing from other jobs as well as a meaningful work culture much like it did for African-American women. Like the dressmaking and millinery trades, hairdressing could also be described in Wendy Gamber's words as "creative labor," seen not simply as a job but rather as a calling in life.[70] As soon as Connolly stepped foot in Mrs. Smith's beauty shop, she knew she wanted to become a beauty operator because in her eyes it seemed so different from the other jobs she had worked in Rochester. Unlike the "old maids" she met around town who never stopped complaining and wore drab clothes day in and day out, Peggy, the head beauty operator, had striking and glamorous red hair. Indeed, when Peggy curled Connolly's hair with an electric curling iron and "piled it high with figure eights," she realized that she too "would love to be an operator on Broadway!" Connolly had grown "weary" of jobs like the one at the hotel, where she was expected to eat alone in the kitchen, enter and exit through the back door, and cater to the demands of less interesting groups of men who cared little for her world of style and romance.[71] And at a time when routinization, time management, and assembly-line work were increasingly popular (among employers), hairdressing promised a highly skilled occupation that defied the larger trends in manufacturing.[72]

Yet rather than undermine the artistry of the occupation, technological changes provided hairdressers with more tools and hence more techniques to master. While women could still manage many of the new styles on their own, increasing numbers of fashion-conscious women found themselves at the mercy of their hairdresser's hands, desperate for a style that was not only the right length, but also the right color and curl. Permanent-wave machines along with an assortment of available dyes demanded training and experience, not to mention someone who knew what concoctions to mix to achieve the desired look. The skill and the artistry of hairdressing, then, meant that it was more than simply a way to make ends meet but something that seemed to blur the distinctions between girlish play and the adult world of work and responsibility. As a girl, Connolly loved to style her hair with a variety of pins, bows, and curls, and she also loved "making dandelion curls," something she insists was rather "prophetic." And even when hairdressing was more work than play, it nevertheless provided an artisanal sense of self rarely associated with the realm of women's wage work. The beauty operator actually created the product in contrast to the department store sales clerk or waitress who sold merchandise. In other words, beauty operators, especially in small neighborhood shops, dominated the labor process from start to finish in a fashion similar to that which labor historians have long insisted was key to worker control, dignity, and pride. In fact, Connolly's dream was not to become just an operator, but in her words an "expert . . . [and] even better, if possible, than Peggy who kept [her] looking so grand."[73]

The beauty shop also afforded women the chance to become entrepreneurs. During the early twentieth century, there was a dramatic increase in "professional jobs" such as teaching and social work as well as office work and retail sales.[74] But while these jobs offered new opportunities for women to work in glamorous stores and brand new office buildings, few were able to enjoy the kind of satisfaction that came from running their own business. As the NHCA noted, beauty shops offered "one of the few opportunities to ambitious women who wish to own their own business."[75] In part, beauty shop ownership reflected the varying degrees of investment needed to open a shop. A pair of scissors, a hot comb, a kitchen sink, along with various solutions to wash, rinse, and change hair color that were either affordable or could be manufactured at home made it relatively easy for some women to set up shops in their own homes or tenement flats. Over time, women could expand their businesses and buy better equipment and furnishings, eventually hiring other operators and on occasion opening another business or two in the same town or city.

Hairdressing also fit neatly into the contours of women's daily lives. Whether one was a worker or a customer, the beauty shop's informality allowed for curlers and combs to intermingle with dishes, diapers, and other domestic duties. After marriage, Connolly "didn't know how two babies could keep one so busy" and admitted that she "went around in a daze most of the time, sterilizing bottles, changing diapers, boiling milk, washing diapers, trying to cook and keep house." Nevertheless, she managed, with the help of "dear Grandmother," to own and operate her own beauty shop and take care of her family's needs. Often located in private homes, beauty shops provided a space for women to earn a living without compromising their daily household responsibilities. Nor did the ability to combine hairdressing and motherhood seem to be a secret. Indeed, at the request of a concerned son,

Connolly promised to help a desperate mother of nine who wanted to learn hairdressing "so that she did not have to work so hard," suggesting that other wage work was either unavailable or far less compatible with a mother's daily regime. And even after children were grown, women remained hairdressers and often grew old with their customers who continued to frequent the shop for the style and company they had claimed as part of their routine, ensuring that the beauty shop would continue to contribute to the family economy throughout a woman's life cycle.[76]

The beauty shop's dramatic growth was also a matter of consumption. Ida Connolly, for example, fell in love with the beauty shop because it offered her an escape from the farm and the chance to recreate herself despite limited resources. Before she ever dreamed of being a beauty operator, she was determined to be a "city girl" and distance herself from what she described as her "farm clumsiness." In the hotel where she first worked, guests arrived from "all over the world" and their style, dress, and speech intrigued Connolly, who dreamed of nothing more than "Clothes, Clothes, Clothes!" and how they might distance her from the manners and mores of the farm life she now found so awkward. As soon as she moved to the city and had "earned sufficient money," she got rid of her "old, dilapidated satchel," her "laced shoes," and her "flour sack underwear made with the imprint still visible." On her occasional visits back to the family farm, she would find her "sisters and the neighbor's girls lying in the grass" dressed in what Connolly described as "their misfit coats and straw hats." In contrast, Connolly "would be dressed up with high-heeled pumps, fitted coat and . . . plume," eager to show off her "new finery," including rouge and perfume she purchased from a local dime store as well as her prized possession— a "silk taffeta changeable dress" with colors that "shone in the sun like a rainbow."[77]

In the early twentieth century, store-bought luxuries like dresses, pumps, and perfume reflected broader changes in women's work that not only provided better wages but more time to enjoy the finer things in life. From 1880 to 1920 the growing trend was toward shorter work days. Increasing numbers of businesses closed early on Saturdays or gave their workers a half-holiday, reducing the average number of hours a day from fourteen to ten nationwide.[78] On the farm by contrast, the only job Connolly could find involved helping a neighbor who was expecting a new baby. The job only paid two dollars a week, and she worked from "dawn until dark" every day of the week. Connolly recalled that she "washed, ironed, cooked, and took care of the little two-year old boy . . . made butter with an old fashioned barrel churn, baked bread for the entire family, and prepared Sunday dinners for uninvited relatives." Once she moved to the city, her day-to-day routine changed dramatically. Connolly explained that she worked hard as a housekeeper at a hotel and later as a waitress, but she had considerably more leisure time than on the farm and more money to spend on fancy dresses, cosmetics, and hair accessories. Connolly was earning eight dollars a week, plus tips and even at the factory, "Sundays and holidays were free."[79]

Getting "all dolled up" was crucial to Connolly's identity as were the dances and dates she now enjoyed on a regular basis. It was, however, the trip to the beauty shop that made her transition from farm to city life complete. Although never as grand as the "palaces of consumption" Susan Porter Benson describes in her study of department stores, beauty shops nevertheless offered women a sense of glamour amidst the most humble surroundings.[80] Besides haircuts and permanent waves, beauticians offered special treatments like facials, manicures, and massages and readily made use of the growing cosmetics industry by offering an array of cosmetics along with hair accessories. Mrs. Smith's Beauty Shop, where Connolly spent much of her free time and money, was a modest establishment located over a bank on Broadway. But to Connolly it seemed a million miles away from the "barny" smells of perspiring farms boys who donned simple overalls to dances, "scooped beans" with a knife, and drank coffee from a "saucer." In the beauty shop, she listened to women's stories about trips across the Atlantic, luxurious ball room dances, and meticulous descriptions of who was wearing what.[81]

Throughout the early twentieth century, changes in style also offered immigrant women the escape for which they may have been looking, especially from their parents and their Old-World traditions. Elizabeth Ewen argues that changes in style and dress were part of the process of breaking from traditional values and becoming more American.[82] In New York in the 1920s, for example, Francisco Bruno, an Italian who immigrated to the United States at the turn of the century, found that his ten daughters were opposed to what he considered traditional values, especially when it came to fashion and style. In a desperate bid "to get the parents' consent to wear their hair like the other girls," his daughters offered "many pleas." But Bruno and his wife remained staunchly opposed to their daughters' desires to bob their hair, until one of them, Dora, "resorted to rebellion." Much to her parents' surprise, she returned home after work "with her hair bobbed." But rather than directly confront her parents, their traditions and authority, Dora offered an elaborate excuse and claimed that "a crazy man in the crowded train must have cut off her hair without her ever becoming aware of the tonsorial operation." Whether or not Bruno and his wife believed Dora, her actions paved the way for her nine sisters, who soon had their hair bobbed just "like the other girls."[83]

Of course, immigrant parents were not the only ones objecting to the new style. According to Connolly, when the bob became popular, "The papers wrote articles about it." "Men lectured on the subject," and "It even became material for one or two sermons."[84] In fact, sensational stories about the bob and the controversy surrounding it proliferated. Men supposedly divorced their wives after having their long locks removed; they often bonded together and refused to shave until their wives agreed to grow their hair out. Women donning the boyish bob also lost jobs in department stores and hospitals while doctors claimed that the bob would eventually lead to the "baldness of the species."[85]

In the 1920s, short skirts, cigarettes, and bobbed hair were also identified with changes in gender and sexual identities. The popularity of the bob in the early twentieth century was accompanied by a growing rejection of the Victorian tenet of self control in favor of what historians have call sexual liberalism—"an overlapping set of beliefs that detached sexual activity from the instrumental goal of procreation . . . [and] defined sexual satisfaction as a critical component of personal happiness."[86] This change, along with increasing opportunities for higher education and new employment, allowed women to step boldly beyond the domestic realm. Christina Simmons argues that as white middle-class women "discarded Victorian delicacy, they seemed more like men, that is, as individuals with a right to personal fulfillment rather than a duty to sacrifice self for men and children."[87] The image of the "new woman" with her bobbed hair was not just a challenge to domesticity, however. In the late nineteenth century, sexologist Richard von Krafft-Ebing associated "homosexual deviance" with the rejection of traditional female roles and cross-dressing. More specifically, he argued that lesbian tendencies "may nearly always be suspected in females wearing their hair short."[88]

Finding a place to have their hair bobbed further encouraged the expansion of the ladies' hairdressing industry. Despite the growing number of hairdressers, there were generally more women demanding to have their hair bobbed than the existing number of beauty shops could handle, a factor that drove many Euro-American women into local barber shops. In New York, it was reported that heads were "being clipped at the rate of 2,000 a day," compelling barber shops to offer quick and easy courses on how to cut the "Boy Bob" to any man's barber. The clamor surrounding the bob was so great in some cities that there were long lines of women outside barber shops while inside women sat on the floor anxiously waiting their turn.[89] And it was not just the adventurous sort. According to one observer, it seemed that "flappers, middle-aged women, even gray-haired grandmothers had invaded man's last retreat, the barber-shop."[90] In Chicago barber shops, one man insisted that "half of the trade" was "composed of women and girls." "If ever the women should decide to quit having their hair cut," this man warned that hundreds of barber shops would be forced to shut their doors.[91]

At the very least, men were ambivalent about this intrusion. When women first began frequenting barber shops, one observer claimed that "old-time barbers rather resented it and seemed to look upon them as intruders." Some of the more experienced barbers even declared that "they would not work in any shop where they were expected to work on women."[92] Barbers did not seem to mind the "few pioneers [who] had bobbed their hair in 1918." But by the early-1920s "women were moving by hordes into the last stronghold of man's privacy——the barbershop."[93] In California, one barber went so far as to place a sign outside his shop that read "FOR MEN ONLY" as if a female clientele would be detrimental to the barber's identity and work culture.[94]

Of course, a female presence was not simply a threat to the barber; men also complained that women were undermining the male culture generally identified with the barber shop. In some cases, the changes were quite subtle. One man, for example, protested that instead of finding *The Sporting Times* or *The Police Gazette* to "pass the time while waiting for the call of 'next,'" he was more likely to pick up *Vogue* or *The Ladies Home Journal*.[95] In other cases, it seemed as if the barber shop had been radically transformed. In 1927, Mrs. W. Y. Morgan, a feature writer for the *Hutchinson* (Kansas News), visited several barbershops and found to her dismay that they were "the dullest experience" of her life. "In the years when for a woman to visit a barber shop was considered the last word in impropriety," she had been taught that "all barber shops were places where interesting conversation went on, and where gossip the like of which a bridge club never dreamed of, took place." Perhaps that had been the case long ago, Morgan thought, but it had "all changed now." Indeed, she was disappointed from the moment she entered the shop. "The first time I seated myself in a barber chair, the man who attended my wants looked and acted more like an undertaker than a glib barber man with a choice bit he was yearning to get out of his system." Much to her dismay, "he discussed the weather at full length." Morgan "didn't know until that day how prolonged the weather topic could be dragged out." And, she continued, "had it not been for a spray of Florida water he shot in my direction— I would never have known I had really been in a man's barber shop."[96]

In hopes of finding more excitement, Morgan sought out several other barber shops, but "all of them have been disappointments—so far as a place for news is concerned." She even began to wonder "how in the world so dull a place as a man's barber shop ever got the reputation of being conversational and spicy." Morgan tried to "get an invitation" to the barbers' state convention, which she thought might "reveal that secret." But her "barber man" looked even "more sad and sorrowful" whenever she "angled for the invitation," leading her to conclude that the nature of barber shops transformed precisely when women "in-

Getting to the Roots of the Industry

vaded" them. Morgan began to think seriously about her female friends' insistence that "the barber men are scared of us." Woefully, she concluded that the "interesting barber shop has slipped into the past, along with long haired women with dragging skirts," implying that the "new woman's" manners and mores had ushered in real and somewhat unwanted changes in men's lives.[97]

Not all barber shops were as tame and refined as Morgan claimed, however. In fact, the barber shop's notorious reputation gave critics one more reason to push for sex-segregated beauty work. Part of that concern about the barber's reputation revolved around the question of his competency. In 1920, the editor of *The American Hairdresser* argued that women should only patronize the beauty shop because "The Beauty Parlor profession in America has risen to a much higher standard than that of the Barber Shop, for we have gone much farther in learning and art." At the same time, the barber's reputation was framed as a question of propriety. The editor reminded the magazine's readers that the beauty shop was designed not only to cater to women, but also to young girls and children and strongly advised that women and children think twice before venturing into the barber shop. "The little girl's patronage especially, because of her sex, of right belongs to the Beauty Parlor, and not to the men's Barber Shop," suggesting that it was little different than the saloon or pool hall.[98] Nine years later in 1929, Mrs. Florence Fay addressed the Ohio State Legislature and demanded laws that would forbid barbers from cutting women's hair. According to *The Journeyman Barber*, Fay insulted the profession because she "insinuated . . . that the barbers were more interested in women's skirts than cutting hair." Fay carefully explained that a woman's modesty was preserved in a beauty shop where a "booth with curtains" surrounded her and the hairdresser, "if it is a man, he stands behind her to cut her hair and not in front of her [like at a barber shop as if] trying to see how short her skirts are."[99]

Barbers' attitudes towards female customers also reinforced concerns about women in barber shops. Many barbers concluded that it was titillation rather than skill that made the barber shop so attractive to women. "Nowadays," insisted one barber, "they [women] demand a good-looking young 'sheik,' one who can 'shoot a good line of bull and jolly the women along.'" One man

44 even argued that "the ability to turn out a first-class haircut is of secondary importance." Some men may "think I am exaggerating," he maintained, "but I can assure them that every word I have said is true, that is, as far as Chicago is concerned." It seemed that "not very long ago," this same barber heard indirectly from the owner of a "fashionable beauty parlor on the North side of Chicago" that one of "her best lady customers . . . did not want any old or middle-aged barber to work on her, as she did not get any 'kick' out of it!" Much to the dismay of the barber, "she liked to have a good-looking young barber do her work, and that she got quite a 'thrill' when a young man handled her hair!"[100]

In cities like Atlanta, where a high percentage of barbers were African-American men, race further complicated concerns over white women's presence in barber shops. Indeed, Euro-American women who had their hair bobbed at the barber shop crossed racially defined gender boundaries and thus violated a long standing taboo against the intermingling of white women and black men. In response, Atlanta's city fathers passed an ordinance that restricted black barbers from cutting white women's hair, something they believed was crucial to the preservation of white female virtue. According to C. Vann Woodward, Atlanta's decision to ban white females from black-owned and operated barber shops tells us much about the pervasiveness of Jim Crow, but it also reveals much about America's hairdressing industry. White Atlanta was well aware of the intimacy between barber and client—the close proximity, the touch, the conversation—the kinds of interactions that seemed most threatening to a city whose economic growth and ideology depended upon racial segregation.[101]

Moreover, in areas where black barbers did not predominate, especially in the northeast, native-born whites were not always the ones to replace them. By the late nineteenth century, southern and eastern Europeans were beginning to displace many African-American service workers, including barbers, doormen, elevator operators, waiters, and cooks, something that Jacqueline Jones argues was "well underway by 1900."[102] Of all the immigrants that arrived between 1899 and 1910 when immigration reached its peak, Italian men, whose own racial identity native-born Americans found suspect, made up nearly 60 percent of im-

bidden space and a threat to white womanhood.[103]

The experience of the beautician herself also reinforced concerns about men's unruly behavior. Just a decade after women invaded barber shops, news headlines described "Males Invading Beauty parlors for Permanents" in what appeared to be a brief reversal in trends as male customers began "flocking to the beauty parlors for their permanents." Nor was it just the sophisticated urbanite. Even "Kansas cow punchers" were found making their way to "beauty shops and salons every spring just before roundups."[104] Of course, men's presence did not always amuse their female operators or the women with whom they shared the beauty shop. Connolly recalled the day a taxi driver brought in a drunken man who demanded a manicure. The other operator "gave one look at him" and refused, but Connolly, feeling that she should do what her "boss asked . . . gave the drunk a manicure." Connolly always remembered how "he looked at me rather maudlin like," called her "girlie," and then much to her dismay began to describe in intimate detail the "awful time" he had been having with his "urination." "I can't urinate!" he declared all too publicly. Expressing her own discomfort, Connolly politely apologized but insisted she could not do anything for him, stating that after all she was "only a beauty operator." Meanwhile, Connolly did not think the conversation appropriate. "I know men had that trouble, but they didn't talk about it in the [beauty] shop."[105]

Other beauty operators may have found these conversations problematic, but they were also particularly aware of the male gaze. In some cases, the beautician simply attracted a lot of unwanted attention. When the marcel wave became popular, Connolly became so busy that she hired another operator named Jenny but every time Jenny worked, a voyeuristic crowd of men was sure to gather outside the beauty shop's front window to watch her every move.[106] In other cases, the beauty operator became the object of sexual fantasy. One Chicago man recalled that as a fifteen year old boy, working in a barber shop shining shoes, he frequently "aroused" his "passion" by walking through "the beauty parlor section of the shop" to catch a glimpse of the manicurist. As the story goes, the "first time" his "sexual passion was aroused," the manicurist was "lying upon the divan reading a magazine" and her "skirt was way above her knees," revealing her "hairy privates." After making several trips through the beauty parlor to the toilet, the head barber became "suspicious" of the boy's behavior. Peeking through a key-hole, the barber caught the boy masturbating. "He told me he was ashamed of me [and] . . . explained to me that if I kept that up I would eventually ruin my health." Giving the boy a dollar, the barber suggested that he "go to the Red Light District around Halstead and Madison." "He gave me the address of a brothel," recalled the former shoe shiner and "told me to mention his name to the land-lady." The barber even "warned me not to the kiss the prostitute, and to be sure and use a contraceptive." More likely than not, the barber had sent other customers to this same land-lady, for the boy was let in despite his youthful age as soon as he mentioned the barber's name.[107]

The struggle over the bob, then, was not simply about the opposition women confronted from men. It was also about male culture. The constant ogling they confronted along with the topics of conversation with which most men amused themselves, the barber shop's link to prostitution, and the fact that women were crossing unfamiliar racial and ethnic boundaries not only gave women several reasons why they might willingly leave the barber shop for their own beauty space but also explains the dramatic expansion of an industry, an industry that developed distinctly along lines of gender.

The barber shop also began to lose favor among many women because they wanted something more than a simple bob: they wanted more complicated services like color and curls. By the 1920s in particular, women not only adopted the boyish bob but also bleached their hair blonde, which contrasted sharply with "one of the striking features of the Victorian model of beauty," namely her dark hair. While the blonde "bombshell" is usually identified with the post-World War II period, she first made her appearance in the 1860s and then reemerged again directly following World War I—when she attracted perhaps as much attention as her more famous post-World War II look alike.[108] For example, in the 1920s, one Italian observer insisted that in Chicago dance halls, gentlemen preferred blondes and showed off their preference by spending more "freely on 'blondes and red-heads' . . . than [on] brunettes."[109] Even at the workplace it appeared that blondes were having more fun, or a least making better tips and wages than their dark-haired counterparts. Dorothy Sue Cobble found that in the 1920s, restauranteurs began experimenting with restaurant decor and began to recognize that restaurant dining could satisfy social and psychological appetites as well. Waitresses, for example, were not only used to serve food but were featured as decorative objects whose presence was designed to enhance the dining experience. In one of New York's most popular restaurants, the management hired attractive waitresses specifically to match the decor. "Service in the Fountainette room is by waitresses with red hair; in the main dining room, blondes; in the lunch room, brunettes," all of which corresponded to a specific hierarchy with blondes and redheads in the more exclusive dining areas where they were likely to receive better tips.[110]

The popularity of blondeness emerged from two different impulses. In her study of hair, sex, and symbolism, Wendy Cooper argues that blondeness and purity were intimately linked.[111] Indeed, psychologist Charles Berg goes so far as to argue that "fair hair . . . [is] less nearly related to the pubic hair" and thus is "taken as symbolic of purity."[112] Hence, blonde hair stood in opposition to hair that was not to be seen and for some contemporaries was crucial to racial purity. In July 1921, Albert Edward Wiggam published "Should I Marry a Blond or Brunette?" in *Physical Culture* and insisted that "'democracy,' 'chivalry' and 'the modern high position' of women will last only 'as long as the blond race lasts.'" He based his arguments on Madison Grant's earlier publication *The Passing of the Great Race* (1916), which warned readers that the "Great Blond Nordic race which has made nearly all modern civilizations is actually being bred out by the lower types of the brunette races."[113] Blondeness was not simply associated with purity, however. Bleached blondes, like other forms of artificial embellishment such as make up and flashy clothes, suggested a more public display of womanhood that was ultimately seen as more sexual, making blondes the epitome of this new public, heterosexual culture. By the 1930s, film star Jean Harlow's platinum-blonde hair had become a trade mark of her sex appeal and set a precedent for the likes of Marlene Dietrich, Jayne Mansfield, Brigette Bardot, and Marilyn Monroe.[114]

While the popularity of blondeness posed obvious contradictions, in that it signified purity in contrast to dark hair and dark skin and embraced a more sensual and sexual self, it also provided women the means to break from a particular past. Blondeness was in fact so closely associated with this new culture of consumption that the dumb blonde emerged simultaneously with the popularity of the new look. According to Wendy Cooper, the "dumb blonde image" was a product of the "frenetic post-World War I period, when the most frivolous of the new flappers were also the most likely to experiment with the platinum blond bleaches."[115] Yet, the dumb blonde may have also been a uniquely ethnic construction. In Anzia Yezierska's autobiographical look at life and love among a Jewish-Russian immigrant family, one sister, Masha, noted for her "golden hair," is nicknamed the "empty head." Almost without thought, Masha readily betrays her family's wishes and traditions in search of this new world of consumption and an American identity:

> Masha worked when she had to work; but the minute she got home, she was always busy with her beauty, either retrimming her hat, or pressing her white collar, or washing and brushing her golden hair. She lived in the pleasure she got from her beautiful face, as Father lived in his Holy Torah.[116]

While Masha's "dumbness" reflected her almost complete and frivolous obsession with her own beauty, the delicate trimming of her hat, and her long and golden hair, her father considered her "empty" or dumb because of her complete rejection of her parents and their immigrant past and traditions.

The ambiguity surrounding blondeness also allowed white men and women to transgress yet reassert certain racial boundaries. Long before advertisers would insist that "blondes have more fun," contemporaries undoubtedly associated blondeness with the make up, the sexually expressive dances, and the footloose and fancy-free attitude associated with the "new woman." But the old adage "blondes have more fun" is problematic. According to bell hooks, it is a "white supremacist assumption" that ignores the "real fun." In other words, the fun which brings "to surface all those 'nasty' unconscious fantasies and longings about contact with the Other embedded in the secret," or as hooks aptly puts it, the "(not so secret) deep structure of white supremacy."[117] By the 1920s, urban areas across the country were feeling the influence of the Great Migration when hundreds of thousands of black men and women packed up their southern belongings and moved north. For example between 1910 and 1920, New York's black population increased by 66 percent and from 1920 to 1930 it increased by 115 percent. The growing black population, Kevin Mumford argues, meant more black/white contacts. On the one hand, the growth of the black population provoked fears about the mixing of the races and led most northern and midwestern states to conduct hearings on antimiscegenation statues. On the other hand, the 1920s became famous as the Jazz Age when young white urbanites went "slumming" at cabarets in Harlem and other black communities and simultaneously embraced, mimicked, manipulated that which they defined as black.[118] Thus the most obvious contradiction: the bleached blonde who embraced an expressive sexuality she identified with black culture may have appeared to transgress racial boundaries yet ultimately she only brought that contradiction into sharper focus, reaffirming her own whiteness and certain assumptions about black culture. The blonde and frivolous flapper might take the A train to Harlem and even adopt black styles of dance, but her blondeness and the kind of "purity" it implied had its own racial overtones that kept her and the men with whom she associated from ever completely crossing the color line.

The permanent wave, which became popular in even out of the way places by the late 1920s and early 1930s further confused racial boundaries. Perming hair like straightening processes, in part, distinguished Euro-American hair care from African-American beauty-culture services. Yet nothing created more controversy than a woman's desire to alter the texture of her hair, something that seemed to tamper a bit too much with racial identity. And in a racially segregated urban milieu, a permanent wave was perhaps the safest way for white women to transgress forbidden racial barriers. If the symbolic importance of hair texture—its straightness or "kinkiness"—is indeed crucial in constructing notions of racial categorization, then white women's desire to "friz" their hair must be understood in terms of their ambivalence surrounding racial identities. Just as blackface meant respectable rowdiness and safe rebellion in antebellum America, perming one's hair, like other forms of racial cross-dressing, allowed white women to flaunt a sense of recklessness yet ultimately retain their own notions of respectability. Like adopting black styles of dance, music, or slang, permed hair created its own style of racial politics.[119]

Changes in style then, were not simply a matter of practicality. The strain of World War I and the demands women confronted at the workplace compelled many of them to adopt their stylish bob. But changes in style were also a question of identity. The rise of a heterosocial and public culture of leisure, the influx of millions of southern and eastern Europeans, the migration of thousands of African Americans, and the emergence of new sexual cultures and identities shattered the conventional boundaries around which women organized their day-to-day lives. The changes in style they adopted only seemed to confirm the changes they faced. At the very least, the boyish cut, the flaxen blonde, and the frizzy hair allowed women to become a central component of this new world of commercial leisure and sexual expressiveness, but only by emphasizing racial and gender difference. While the bobbed look called into question the often rigid gender divisions that separated men from women, a more sexually expressive look and feel that emphasized the flapper's femininity along with make up and fancy dresses accompanied it. And while the blonde bomb-shell of the period allowed women to project a more sexually expressive demeanor, her platinum look stood in bold contrast to the black hair and darker skin of the southern and eastern Europeans who were immigrating to this country and the men and women with whom she consorted at cabarets and other commercial amusements.

Throughout the first two decades of the twenty century, African-American and Euro-American women defined what the beauty shop meant to individual women by the ways in which they used their businesses. For many women, the beauty shop offered them the homosocial space they needed to forget, at least temporarily, the problems they faced at home and at the workplace or the free space they needed to collectively devise strategies to confront them. Indeed, operators went to great lengths to cultivate and maintain a clientele, ensuring a livelihood that contrasted sharply with domestic work and other forms of wage work all the while promoting the development of an all-female culture.

The beauty shop did, of course, insist upon certain racial and gender boundaries. On the one hand, men and women often found the culture of men they confronted in barber shops offensive, and barbers had neither the expertise nor the experience to handle much more than a bob not to mention the perm machine or the chemicals needed to perfect the platinum blonde look. On the other hand, white women helped define an occupation that stood in opposition to the black hair-care industry. The vision of womanhood they embraced might have offered a much more sexually expressive look than their Victorian counterparts, but it also reinforced the racial boundaries white America was desperately trying to enforce. Indeed, the links between style, race, and identity were so completely intertwined that by the 1930s, Gladys Porter and her San Antonio school mates could not even conceive of a beauty business that catered to both black and white customers. And even if they could, it was not the work culture of which they wished to be a part.

Despite differences between African-American and Euro-American beauty shops, they were nevertheless part of the same history that provided a silent yet ever present connection to a broader political economy. Whether beauticians were curling hair or straightening it, they faced similar challenges. While the beauty shop may have served as a retreat for female customers, it was a job characterized by long hours and low wages for beauticians. In fact, beauticians, regardless of the communities in which they worked, often shared a common sense of disillusionment as they struggled to survive both the unregulated growth of the industry during the 1920s and the Great Depression.

2

Beauty School Promises and Shop Floor Practices

In 1933, Lucille Miller, of Cleveland, Ohio, had worked as a beauty operator for fifteen years and considered her "judgement" of the industry to be "fair" and "reliable." According to Miller, "operators do the hardest manual labor continually using their arms, shoulders, [and] hands—in scrubbing dirty heads, (and God knows they are dirty) marcelling, permanent waving [not] to mention some of the ordinary work of an all around [operator]." Miller explained that the beauty operator also had to answer phones, make appointments, and greet customers, all as she tried "to please the customer she is working on." After twelve hours in a beauty shop, Miller insisted, anyone would be "a total wreck-mentally & physically."[1]

As Lucille Miller voiced her concerns, she exposed an inherent contradiction in the industry: A beauty operator was to act like a professional even though she was treated like an unskilled worker. Moreover, "An operator (a good one)," argued Miller, "spends from two hundred dollars to five hundred" on her education while a "typist, stenographer, file clerk and many other employees in offices get most [of] their training in high school at no additional cost." But after attending beauty schools and paying exorbitant tuitions to become licensed professionals, beauty operators stood on their feet all day and worked "longer hours for less pay than unskilled factory workers."[2] To be sure, women found more affordable ways to learn beauty culture. Public schools and apprenticeship often provided the skills and training women needed to enter the profession. At the same time, however, the Labor Advisory Board's investigation of the beauty industry supported Miller's complaints about long hours and low wages. The Board claimed that various beauty schools, including one in New York which used a "success story" entitled "From Factory Worker to Beautician," needed to rethink their advertising schemes if they wanted to continue to attract students willing to pay such hefty fees.[3]

Despite the Labor Advisory Board's skepticism, beauty school enrollment continued to rise throughout the 1920s and even during the Depression. The Board concluded that increasing enrollment reflected a lack of alternatives on the part of women, but it was more than desperation that attracted women to the field of beauty culture.[4] Throughout the 1920s and 1930s beauticians faced a highly unorganized industry that simultaneously created obstacles and opportunities. On the one hand, beauty shops frequently failed to come under the jurisdiction of protective labor legislation, which meant that beauticians such as Lucille Miller did indeed work longer days for less pay than many "unskilled" factory workers.[5] On the other hand, this lack of regulation afforded women, even with the most meager resources, the chance to turn their flats into makeshift beauty shops and themselves into pink collar professionals and entrepreneurs. Similarly, countless numbers of women, many of whom had little or no formal training in beauty culture, travelled door-to-door "pressing" hair or putting in finger waves, enabling them to make ends meet even during the toughest of times.

Confronting both limitations and possibilities as women in the beauty-culture industry, beauty operators sought to challenge the contradictions they found endemic to their trade. During the early years of the beauty business, operators faced a number of uncertainties that challenged their skills, their emotions, and their customers' sensibilities on a day-to-day basis. Everything from untested hair dyes and equipment to changes in the weather affected the daily operation of beauty shops, conditions compounded by the declining economy of the late 1920s. In order to gain greater control over this highly unregulated industry and create a more favorable work culture, beauticians offered their clients a variety of services that went well beyond a stylish coiffure. Above all, social interactions, which led to lasting relationships between customers and operators, provided opportunities for operators to effectively negotiate wages, hours, and working conditions. Although other service workers such as saleswomen and waitresses also relied on customer loyalty to negotiate a more favorable work environment, the intensity of the operator-client relationship in beauty shops was hard to match. In her study of dressmakers and milliners, Wendy Gamber argues that helping patrons with their "psychological and emotional needs—was integral to the production of women's clothing." This was even more true in the beauty industry. Hairdressers' relationships with their clients often lasted a lifetime and profoundly shaped the nature of work culture and worker resistance as operators struggled to make beauty school promises come true.[6]

By the late 1920s and 1930s, the hairdressing industry was no longer just trying to simply establish itself, but competing against the growing field of white-collar work and trying to fashion a sense of respectability associated with teaching, social work, and especially nursing.[7] Influenced by the trend toward professionalism, industry leaders along with many beauty schools urged the adoption of "such terms as beautician, cosmetition, cosmetologist, cosmetic therapist" in order to legitimize their trade and justify high tuition fees.[8] In particular, beauty schools attempted to out do other female-dominated occupations by promising students a career in beauty culture that would provide financial independence and security for themselves and their families. E. Burnham's School of Beauty Culture in New York and Chicago provided prospective students rags-to-riches stories. One beauty school graduate, for example, was described as a "widow," who found in "Burnham's the means of independence" and a chance to educate her children, while a forty-five year old waitress "without even a grade school education" managed to become the manager of a large beauty shop in just six months after graduation. Perhaps the most remarkable success story told the tale of "a foreign girl seemingly destined solely for work in a factory," who in as little as three years owned four beauty shops and went from "$15.00 a week in a factory to over $10,000.00 a year."[9]

Beauty schools also tried to impress the families of potential students who would presumably help pay tuition fees. "Thinking fathers, nowadays," insisted Burnham's, should "encourage their daughters who want to engage in a money-making activity," because "they know that in so doing they are contributing to their daughters' happiness and welfare." Burnham's even warned parents that all a daughter who lacks marketable skills "can hope for is work in an office or factory, clerking in a store, ushering in a theater, or something else equally ill-paid and devoid of a future." Burnham's continued to explain that "a girl going into such occupations is simply marking time."[10] Similarly, the Wilfred Academy, which had branches in several East Coast cities, argued that beauty culture was the best choice for any woman regardless of her background. "Beauty culture," Wilfred's claimed, was an "easy and natural occupation, inherent in practically all women," emphasizing a woman's supposed affinity for grooming, beauty, and style.[11]

Being a professional meant more than money, however; it meant expertise. In an attempt to live up to their promises, beauty schools offered a wide variety of courses designed to teach every aspect of the business. The New York State Department of Labor, for example, found that "For the girl without previous training or experience who wishes to become a general operator in a beauty shop, most of the schools offer complete courses to fit her for any type of work an operator might be required to do." The vast majority of the workers in beauty shops were known as general operators or "all-round girls" and were trained in a variety of beauty treatments. Many schools offered standard courses in shampooing and hairdressing and classes that taught the art of marcelling, finger waving, water waving, permanent waving as well as dying and bleaching, services common to most shops. Some schools also gave lectures and demonstrations in manicuring and scalp and facial treatment, including "electrical treatments with vibrators and violet rays, muscle strapping and beauty packs."[12] At Burnham's one would not simply learn to do hair but master "methods" and "techniques" from a well-trained "faculty" who provided students with lectures, demonstrations, and practical experience in all types of styles and techniques.[13] And the instruction was often on an individual basis, with students practicing on models, on each other, and even on the instructor. Eventually, students would work on customers at reduced rates or free of charge. In general, the "larger" schools provided their students with text books to supplement the occasional lecture, and a few schools featured "elementary business courses" and "lectures on the psychology of running a shop."[14]

To further enhance its reputation beauty schools also offered courses that blurred distinctions between beauty culture and professions like medicine. Many schools provided what they classified as "scientific" instruction, including "lectures on anatomy and physiology and instruction in the principles of sanitation and sterilization."[15] The Wilfred Academy featured facial beauty courses in which students not only learned how to apply "Street and Evening Make-up" but were also taught how to treat "Course Pores, Blackheads, Freckles, [and] Acne," as well as what instructors called "Cosmetic defects." In an electrolysis course, for example, students learned the "most scientific method used for removing Superfluous Hair . . . [with] the Multiple Needle Method." Another course entitled "Scientific Fundamentals" focused on "the principles and methods of Sterilization, Sanitation, and Hygiene," while lectures were given on the "Anatomy and Physiology of the Skin." Wilfred's also expected students to learn about human hair's natural growth patterns and diseases as well as aspects of the muscular, circulatory, and nervous systems.[16] Similarly, Burnham's beauty-culture students spent hours "studying nerves, circulation, the structure of the skin, the metabolism of the cells, [and] functions of the different muscles connected with beauty culture." Many beauty schools also featured photos of teachers and students dressed in nurses' uniforms bent over what appeared to be patients rather than the typical beauty shop patron.[17] And, according to Lois Banner, beauty parlors "generally had white, enamelled furniture to give them the hygienic look of hospitals to boost the beauty operator's claims of scientific expertise."[18]

Promises of professionalism and economic well-being undoubtedly tempted some women to invest in the most prestigious schools, yet convenience, affordability, and location were also important considerations. Rural areas and small towns generally lacked their own beauty schools because of the smaller pool of students from which to draw. And if there were enough potential students, there was usually only one school. North Platte, Nebraska, for example, had a population of 12,069 in 1934, a population large enough to support twenty-five beauty shops but only one school.[19] In contrast, large urban areas offered prospective students a number of options. A 1931 investigation of New York revealed an abundance of beauty schools that varied greatly according to size, tuition, and location. The city boasted approximately eighty beauty schools, the vast majority of which had been established since the early 1920s. While some schools were quite large with space for 100 students and attracted more than 500 students each year, others seldom had more than 10 students at a time. Investigators noted that many of the larger schools had "attractive quarters" and "modern beauty parlor equipment," while they described others as "dingy," "poorly equipped," and not so different from the "poorest type of cut-rate beauty shop." Moreover, many of these "poorly equipped" schools were considered to be "short-lived" establishments, especially since they were "not even listed in the classified telephone directory."[20]

Tuition fees and degree requirements also varied considerably. In general, tuition fees ranged from seventy-five dollars to two hundred and fifty dollars for courses that lasted anywhere from six weeks to six months. In addition to the commercial schools, many public schools offered free courses such as the Manhattan Industrial High School for Girls, the Manhattan Evening Trade School, and the Bronx Industrial High School for Girls. Even the Young Women's Christian Association provided training in beauty culture, "at fees somewhat lower than those charged by the average commercial school."[21]

The proliferation of beauty schools, however, even in smaller towns and cities suggests that beauty schools were becoming an industry in and of themselves. This was in part because beauty culture classes were not consistently offered in public schools or that women often found the beauty school a quicker way to reach their occupational goal. Frequently labeled "diploma mills," some schools were often blamed for adding poorly trained operators to an already overcrowded job market, especially by the 1930s.[22] "When I learned this business some years ago," noted Daisy Schwartz, a beautician from New York, "I paid no less than two hundred and fifty dollar's and went to school for 9 months. But today the schools' are turning out unfit workers in two to six weeks time and taking a hundred dollars from these same people."[23]

Beauty school owners were also criticized for using cheap student labor to undercut "legitimate" shop prices. This was especially the case with smaller towns where a single beauty school not only produced fierce competition among beauty shops but also exacerbated larger class-based tensions in the community. Elizabeth Gideon, owner of Fairdame Beauty Shop in North Platte, Nebraska, where there were twenty-five shops and one school complained that the school charged students fifty-five dollars for tuition and undercut the other shops with "special permanents $1.00, $1.50 and $2.00. Marcels 25c, fingerwaves 15c and 25c." To make matters worse, some of North Platte's wealthier citizens spent their beauty dollars at the school instead at one of the town's beauty shops. According to Gideon, "We are spending our money with business men, doctors and dentists, paying their prices and their wives are going to the school for cheap work." "You would be surprised to know how many businessmen's wives, doctors wives, [and] lawyers' wives, who have plenty, patronize this school."[24] Some shop owners even argued that schools should be prevented from serving the general public. For example, in the early 1930s, Mabel English Sanders, owner of The Elite Beauty Shoppe, had been a beautician for twenty-five years and was "one of the oldest, if not the oldest shop owners in Savannah [Georgia]." Sanders, who also suffered from beauty school competition, suggested that rather than undercutting shop owners by offering cheap prices to the public, beauty schools should use children from "orphanages for students to practice on."[25]

School owners, of course, defended their establishments by arguing that their schools were not geared toward the wealthy but instead designed to serve the needs of working-class women by providing both an affordable education and reasonably priced services. Small beauty school owner Betty Jean of Mansfield, Ohio, claimed that

The elimination of the charge for beauty work done in the school and the consequent closing down of hundreds o[f] Beauty Schools will increase the average tuition fee of Beauty Culture, and will automatically bar the girl of small means from learning the beauty culture profession and will deprive her of earning her livelihood therefrom.

Betty Jean further insisted that "charging a small amount to the public [for] beauty service given by the students brings down the cost to the student for tuition." Women "who patronize the Beauty Schools are in the main from the poorer and working classes," she declared. And they "cannot afford to pay the prices asked by regular beauty shops during normal times." Preventing beauty schools from serving the general public, she claimed, "would deprive this multitude of women of the poorer classes, shop girls, and domestics, who look to the beauty schools for their beauty work, of the opportunity that they now possess of beautifying themselves at very little expense."[26]

Of course even if schools were able to offer reasonable tuition rates, many women who wanted to learn the trade got their start and training as an apprentice. During the early years of the beauty shop, some operators hired apprentices who, in exchange for working in the shop, learned the art of hairdressing. By the 1930s, the practice seemed to be waning, especially among the larger New York shops, which refused to employ "beginners with neither training nor experience." The decline of the practice was a welcome change for investigators who argued that "this type of training" was "unsatisfactory," because "the proprietor teaches the girl in spare moments; there is no definite plan of instruction." But in the face of the Depression, small New York shops contin- ued to hire apprentices as they could no longer afford to hire "reg- ular operators," and they often needed the training fee. In some of the shops students exchanged their labor for instruction while other shops charged the apprentice any where from thirty-five dollars to one hundred dollars.[27] According to Emily Weber of the Labor Advisory Board, apprenticeship was highly contested be- cause in "many localities" wages were being "undermined" be- cause of the "practice of employing large numbers of so-called 'learners' . . . at unbelievably low wages or at no wages at all, only to discharge them at the end of this 'learning' period to be re-placed by another group of the same type."[28]

In fact, despite continued opposition to the apprenticeship sys-tem, it was still in place in some communities as late as the 1950s. Louise Long, for example, started to learn the art of beauty cul-ture when she was "ten or twelve" from her cousin who during the 1950s owned a shop that catered exclusively to African-Amer-ican women in the small mid-Missouri town of Mexico. Long re-called that when the "sisters [her cousins] were fixing hair, then we would kind of clean up the hair on the floor while they cut the hair." And once everyone "left we would wash the basin, wash the mirror and clean up the whole shop so it would be ready for the next day [and] sometimes we could go there on Saturdays and she would have us dusting." But Long still found time to learn the trade. "You see as I was working in my cousins' shop I would watch them . . . I was suppose to be working, but I would slow down to watch them to see what they were doing." Before long she started practicing on herself "and the next thing I knew I was just pressing and curling. It wouldn't take me just fifteen minutes to press and fifteen minutes to curl." Once "I got good at it," Long explained, "I had everybody in Mexico, coming to my house," with as many as eighteen customers coming "on a regular basis."[29]

Besides the apprenticeship system, women who lacked other opportunities or the wherewithal to pay for beauty school simply taught themselves. In the fall of 1925, Mrs. Leland Everett Hall of Athens, Illinois opened her own beauty shop, but only after she taught herself the tricks of the trade. Her brother Ray, a barber, initially piqued her interest in the occupation by asking her point blank, "why in the world don't you start marcelling?" Going to beauty school had never crossed her mind, and Hall did not "know anything about" the beauty business. But Ray eventually convinced her to visit "Ruthie Horn over in Mason City," because "she's doing real good" in the business. Ray also bought his sister "a curling iron and a heater," reassuring her that "there's nothing to it." "All you have to do," he said, "is stick that iron in there and pull on it," and "if you turn it over it just makes the prettiest curls." Hall was a bit reluctant and worried about what might "happen when you turn that iron on." So she decided to take some lessons from Ruthie Horn, who showed her a few things, but never really taught her how to handle the iron. Instead, Hall experimented on her own with "a piece of hair" that she had nailed to the "back of an old kitchen chair." After hours of standing in front of that "old kitchen chair," she gradually "figured on her own" just how to hold the comb, the iron, and that "piece of hair." Then she practiced on neighbors and friends, curling "hair up one side and down the other," free of charge, until she knew she could "do it right." It was not too long before practice made perfect and she had a steady stream of paying customers as well as a successful beauty shop in her very own home.[30]

Despite success stories like Ruth Hall's, the dramatic growth of the industry throughout the 1920s and 1930s compelled an increasing number of states to pass cosmetology laws, demanding that beauty operators meet specific educational requirements. These laws lacked any uniformity, however. In 1931, for example, laws concerning the amount of formal training beauticians were required to have for licensing varied dramatically from state to state. Some states, such as Connecticut, demanded that operators obtain a minimum of 2,100 hours of training spread out over a year, while Nevada required only 400 hours. Seventeen states required an eighth grade grammar school education, while four states had no preliminary educational requirement. In fact, only twenty-four states and one territory had any minimal requirements at all. Much to the dismay of *The American Hairdresser*, only five states east of the Mississippi passed any cosmetology legislation; two New England states, Connecticut and Rhode Island, had laws regarding licensing but none of the mid-Atlantic states did.[31]

Because of a lack of any minimal requirements and the high demand for training in beauty culture, beauty schools began to establish their own restrictions. Nearly half of all New York City's beauty schools required that students be at least fourteen years old, occasionally a student had to be sixteen or even eighteen. At the same time, some schools demanded that students satisfy a minimum educational requirement, even though an education was "considered of little importance in beauty shop work."[32] Instead, an education was valued primarily because it gave future employees the "added poise" they needed "to talk more intelligently with customers." "A good education may be an advantage" investigators noted, but only "to a girl seeking work in a first class shop." Regardless of her skills, finding work in a Fifth Avenue shop meant the right dress and manners. Above all, beauty schools, like prospective employers, expected students to possess an "attractive personality," "good complexions," shapely "figures," and in general "look the part."[33]

Industry leaders were never that clear about what "looking the part" exactly meant, but throughout the 1920s and 1930s the most profound restrictions in the hairdressing industry continued to fall along lines of race, and beauty schools were no exception. Although schools were looking for operators with shapely figures, they usually accepted male students. But only half of those in New York accepted African-American women and, in these cases, students usually received "individual instruction outside of class." As a result, most African-American women attended black-owned schools. In Harlem, investigators found "a number [of] schools in beauty culture for Negro operators," which were often connected to "large 'systems'" that had their own chains of shops and schools in various cities and "which manufacture beauty preparations for Negro women and equipment for shops which have adopted their methods."[34] Many of these "large systems" were undoubtedly connected to branches of Annie Turnbo Malone's Poro College and Madame C. J. Walker's company.

African-American beauty shops also offered a "somewhat" different set of services than Euro-American businesses. While beauty operators who served a white clientele found that their largest revenue came from permanent waves to create soft shoulder-length curls popular in the 1930s, African-American women had their hair straightened in a process known as "pressing or refining," which was usually given in combination with a shampoo. The Women's Bureau found shampooing and pressing to be a "slow process," taking "more than an hour, sometimes as much as two hours." After the hair was pressed, marcels were given— "beautifully arranged coiffures of smooth and pleasing waves." The entire process needed to be repeated after every shampoo and in hot and humid conditions even more frequently. Like their Euro-American counterparts, African-American women considered themselves "all-around" operators even though hair press-

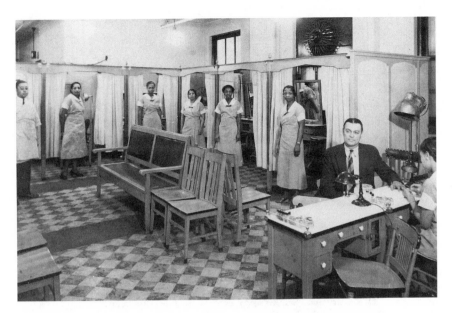

Madame C. J. Walker Beauty Shop, South Center Department Store, Chicago, c. 1940. Courtesy of Vivian G. Harsh, Collection of Afro-American History and Literature, Carter G. Woodson Regional Library, Chicago, Ill., Marjorie Stewart Joyner Collection.

ing and shampooing were the "main source of revenue" in black-owned shops. With the exception of the most expensive shops, which might offer facials and manicures, African-American beauty shops generally provided fewer services than small white-owned neighborhood shops, which almost always featured shampooing, finger waving, haircutting, and manicuring.[35] In New Orleans, for example, The Moro Beauty Shop, owned by Mrs. W. Kile, employed five "hair pressers," who offered customers a "shampoo and press combined for 25c." According to the Women's Bureau, "it was the only service" the shop "offered to an appreciable extent." In fact, investigators doubted that any other services were given. "The better type of shop" charged seventy-five cents for the same service, with a slight discount for customers who came on a regular basis, usually every other week.[36]

However a woman acquired the training to be a successful beautician, once she found a job, she entered a world even more

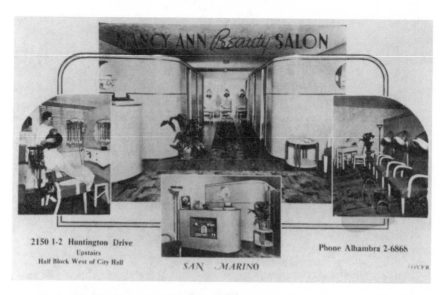

Postcard featuring "San Marino's Most Modern Beauty Salon," owned by Nancy Ann Hamilton, c. 1935. Courtesy of Ann Howe.

diverse than that of beauty-culture education. In Manhattan, for example, the New York Department of Labor found beauty shops that occupied "several floors of a modern office building" and employed as many as seventy-five to one hundred operators. These large shops, investigators noted, "provided conspicuous examples of the expansion of the beauty culture industry." Cities also boasted "large" beauty shops in department stores and "fashionable" hotels.[37] For example, East Coast elegance was defined in terms of style, modernity, and grandeur. "Royal's newest beauty shop," which was part of the largest chain on Long Island, opened its fourth shop in Jamaica, New York. Royal's provided its patrons with a "luxurious reception room" and "forty-four booths, exquisitely appointed according to the newest ideas in beauty shop construction." Each booth and partition were made from "genuine walnut" and "equipped with a handsome display case, containing a full line of cosmetics." Similarly, in Wilmington, Delaware, The Cohn Beauty Parlor offered the "most attractive modernistic design of black and silver with accessories of tangerine red." The rooms were "large and airy," and "Mirrors are hung about the waiting room to catch the light and reflect it," while lamps added an extra feature to the "color scheme."[38]

Despite the elegance generally associated with the larger and more expensive shops, the fancier businesses did not necessarily provide beauty operators with a more favorable work environment. For example, such shops were likely to have more rigid dress codes than the small neighborhood shop, something many beauty operators protested. Lucille Miller explained that "an operator (if she be employed in an exclusive shoppe) must buy two sets of uniforms twice [a] year (spring and fall) and launder them herself, because as a rule they are too fine and delicate to send to the laundry."[39] Even more intrusive were managerial inspections. In Chicago, employees of The Powder Box faced a stringent dress code and bi-weekly inspections. All employees were dressed in "a soft rose and green combination," noted Betty Jane Harding, Powder Box's manager. "By its uniform we have distinguished each group of workers and at the same time maintained color harmony throughout the salon." "The operators," she continued to describe, "wear rose and the desk girls green, while our maids are dressed in regulation black and white." Harding insisted that in order "to maintain a high standard of appearance, even in a small shop, there must be some system of inspection. We have a regular inspection twice weekly." Not only were the uniforms expected to appear "fresh," but "should uniforms become unduly soiled" while shampooing or doing "dye work," employees must "change at once." Similarly, "the condition of the hair, skin and nails of the operator should always be beyond criticism." In order to "inspire the confidence" of customers who then might be convinced to spend their money in the salon, management expected operators to appear literally without a hair out of place. "We do not allow an operator to appear with a finger-wave that has not been properly combed nor to work with a net over her head." Nor was there any room for excuses. "Beauty services," asserted Harding, were "free to employees in the shop, and there is no reason why they should not take the fullest advantage."[40]

The Powder Box's emphasis on the appearance of its operators and other service workers may have "inspired the confidence" of women unsure about any change in their own style and looks. But the dress codes and other rules also granted managers greater

66

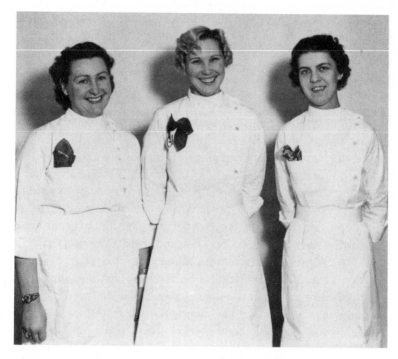

Nancy Ann Hamilton (center) and two employees dressed to perfection and not a hair out of place, c. 1935. Courtesy of Ann Howe.

control over the shop floor and reaffirmed class distinctions. While the shop's rules insisting that hair be properly combed and nails polished ensured a level of respectability among its employees, which undoubtedly made its middle-class clients more comfortable, the dress codes established a rigid hierarchy that made it easier for customers to distinguish between different service workers and maintain an obvious amount of social distance between themselves and the women who served them.

Of course, most women did not have to face the picky rules and restrictions associated with the fancier shops, since most beauticians either owned their own business or worked in a small shop with one or two operators. According to Cincinnati shop owner Murray Kane, beauty shops were divided into "four classes." First, there were salons in department stores, which "were usually controlled by one of four eastern syndicates, who lease the de-

Beauty School Promises and Shop Floor Practices

partment on a percentage basis and operate at huge profits as they 67
have the good will of the department store and a ready made
clientele." Second, there was the "average beauty shop" located
in an office building with one or two operators. According to
Kane, "thousands of these shops are opened and closed constantly." Third, he described shops like his own—"the large advertised beauty shops who take the best downtown, main floor
locations, who keep plenty of operators busy at prices which
meet the popular demand, pay real rents and thousands of dollars
in equipment and advertising." Fourth, there were "hundreds of
girls who graduate from some beauty school, open a shop at their
homes, charge practically nothing for their work, and only create
hardship for the legitimate shop owner."[41]

While Murray challenged the legitimacy of the small neighborhood shops, others claimed that the make-shift shop located in
or outside the home formed the mainstay of the industry. The vice
president of an Illinois Hairdressing Association insisted that
"the vast majority" of beauty shops were "small, independent
shops, employing none, or only a few operators." These shops, he
continued, were "the backbone of the Industry and collectively
employ more operators" than the other groups combined, embracing about 75% of the 50,000 shops and 300,000 persons engaged in Beauty Culture."[42] In New York, for example, so-called
"bath-room" beauty shops were everywhere, tucked away in the
crowded tenements and unused business space.[43] Indeed, investigators agreed that New York shops were generally small and employed only a few operators. In the Bronx, for example, beauty
parlors "with from one to three workers" were "the most common." The majority of these shops were "located on business
streets [and] in stores and office buildings," while others were in
"apartment houses and tenements, a few in old wooden buildings." In Brooklyn, beauty parlors were usually located on the
first floor of stores or office buildings, although there were "a few
in old wooden buildings" and some in the owner's apartments or
some other tenement. A few of these shops were "small and
crowded, with poor lighting and ventilation" or were "dirty and
in bad condition." Even in Manhattan, where investigators found
during the slack season three shops with as many as seventy-five
employees, those that were owner-operated were still the "most

Beauty School Promises and Shop Floor Practices

common." Also in Queens, the average shop hired one employee, and in Brooklyn and the Bronx, the average number of workers per shop was two. In Harlem, investigators insisted that it was "fairly common" to find African-American women operating beauty shops in their own homes. In fact, the majority of African-American beauty operators "work independently" no doubt because of the greater sums of capital needed to set up a beauty shop and to hire other operators and because of the fewer resources black women had to spend on their beauty needs.[44]

In fact even when they worked independently, African-American women did not necessarily own their own shops. As Jacqueline Jones argues, many African-American beauty operators worked on an "informal basis, often in their own homes or in small rented booths in a store."[45] According to the Women's Bureau, "booth rental" was especially common among African-American beauty operators. "Instead of having a whole room or more at their disposal, for a stipulated sum—$2 or $3 a week—a booth, a chair, a shampoo board, or other equipment, together with light and hot water, are rented." Many women opened their first business in their homes and only after developing a steady clientele would they rent a shop. In order to pay the rent, however, they would sublet part of the shop or a booth to other beauty operators. In fact, some shop owners rented space to "their superior operators rather than take the risk of these operators opening competing shops and thus taking trade from the original proprietors." Booth-renting in a well-established shop also made it easier for many women to enter the profession. The Women's Bureau insisted that booth-renting offered just as much flexibility and independence as proprietorship because "They have their own customers and arrange their hours and appointments," and there was less risk involved and less capital to invest.[46]

Countless numbers of beauty operators also went door-to-door, either paving the way to "respectability" or simply making ends meet. African-American entrepreneur, Mrs. Emma Shelton, owned the first beauty shop in Winona, Minnesota. According to a former employee, Evelyn (Peterson) Bambenek, Shelton "started her career walking with her satchel to her customers around town to shampoo their hair." Thanks to a wealthy and steady white clientele, Shelton eventually opened her own shop and offered a variety of services, ranging from hair treatments and massages to corn and callous removal. "She and her shop were well known in the Winona area," Bambenek recalled. Besides offering the "best in hair treatment and massage" to "Winona's upper class," Shelton also provided food to the needy. "Many bums would stop at the shop," remembered Bambenek, and "Mrs. Shelton would always call the restaurant around the corner to give this person a bowl of soup."[47] In addition, African-American women who served exclusively a black clientele often made very little money pressing hair. Hair pressers generally worked "either in their own kitchens where they press hair for 25 cents, or by carrying pressing oil and irons from house to house to ply their services in the homes of customers." When times were hard, hair pressers sometimes worked in exchange for food or other necessities. According to the Women's Bureau, "this itinerant type of service was the bane of the regular shop owners and many disparaging tales were told about it," including examples "of women bartering hair-pressing for food, clothing, or anything else of use to them."[48]

Bartering, however, should not be ignored or dismissed as merely a "disparaging tale." Similar exchanges of goods and services were an everyday experience for many working people and something that became increasingly common even in well-established beauty shops during the Depression. "I saw every phase of the depression in my shop," remembered Ida Connolly. "One dry spell, when there was no feed for cows, one of my customers fed leaves to her only cow and sold the cream to get money for her permanent." Connolly also remembered how "customers often came in with shoes dusty from hitch-hiking their way into town, some as many as twenty miles."

> Many had torn linings in their coats. They couldn't pay more than three dollars for a permanent. Some could not pay at all, but traded things for it. I guess I started a regular trading post, because I traded things for most anything; canned fruits and vegetables, potatoes, chickens, pillows, quilts and fancy-work.

Once, Connolly recalled, a "proud man" brought in a "hand crocheted bedspread" and quietly asked "about trading the spread for a permanent wave for [his] wife," who apparently "was in poor health." Another "man did some painting" for Connolly "to pay for his wife's permanent." One of the most unusual requests came when "an elderly woman came into the shop and asked, 'Could you help me by letting me use [a] little electricity?'" She had an electric toaster under her arm and just wanted "to make a couple of slices of toast." "'Go right ahead,' I said, and she went away happy." But Connolly did not just "take from the community." In the back of her shop, she also kept clothes she picked up at rummage sales, which she then "gave out to people who needed them."[49]

Of course the beautician did have to make a living even as their customers faced the hardest of times. "Business slumped, and we hardly knew just what to do," recalled Connolly. "I spent many hours talking to customers about prices. One woman, I remember well, had only ten dollars to buy a new dress, a pair of shoes and also [to] get a permanent wave." It was also increasingly common to hear customers ask "May I charge my permanent?" Sometimes even "a perfect stranger" would stop by the shop and ask to take out a loan, something on which Connolly had to draw the line. "When money was scarce in those days," even regular customers might try to scam a free permanent. "One day a customer, Mrs. Phillips, came in and insisted that her 'permanent didn't stay.'" After checking her records, Connolly discovered that it had been seven months since Mrs. Phillips' last visit, and her permanent had simply "grown out in that time." Mrs. Phillips would not take no for an answer, however. "Perhaps you made a mistake in your files," she protested, an accusation Connolly thought "was going a bit too far."[50]

Difficult customers were not simply a product of hard times, however. "Every job serving the public has many sides," insisted Connolly, and the beauty shop was "no exception." After Connolly "began to get steady customers," she realized how difficult it was to please "such a wide range of personalities." Connolly's clientele were mostly working girls, school teachers, and clerks. Yet, "It was hard to suit them all." The first time a customer complained that "She didn't buff my nails enough," Connolly was reduced to tears.[51] In 1924, *The Beautician*, a trade journal, defined the "tough customer" as an "unreasonable individual who enters your establishments without knowing what she wants" yet still "expects to have it handed to her on a golden platter." A problem customer, the article continued to describe, "resents every advance made by your attendants to serve her, flies off the handle though you handle her with kid gloves, becomes sarcastic, even downright mean." Nor did the complaining customer respect the operators. Instead, she "marches right up to the beauty general [manager]" because "she wouldn't dream of bringing a complaint to a mere operator!," suggesting that class distinctions could exacerbate customer-client relations.[52]

Beauticians also frequently complained about the condition of some of their less fortunate clients. Once a year, Connolly dreaded the return of a man who brought his wife into the shop for an annual clean up. Her hair was always "matted to her head" and "full of stick-tights and burdocks." Connolly remembered spending hours, using "shampoo, vinegar, alcohol, scissors, and my manicure instruments to pick it, bit by bit, into strands I could comb."[53] "Our work isn't always pleasant," insisted Mary Triella, of Dover, New Jersey, "not when we have to serve an inferior class of people who think only of beautifying [the] top of [their] head while their scalp is 'filthy' or diseased."[54] But *The Beautician* reminded operators that even in the most unpleasant situations, one should always be tactful. "You can't tell her [the customer] that the texture of her hair is like a collie's." Instead, blame it on the weather, "pacifying her . . . by reminding her that the atmosphere has been exceptionally humid during the last few days." If a beautician found a scalp in a "deplorable state—dry, lots of dandruff, hair scant and brittle, suggest a series of scalp treatments, and special shampoos" which over time would lead to a healthier head of hair.[55]

Masking one's emotions was, of course, not unique to the beauty business. In her study of flight attendants, Arlie Russell Hochschild argues that service workers often fall victim to what she calls "emotional labor," in that they have to suppress their true feelings "in order to sustain the outward countenance that produces the proper state of mind in others."[56] Like flight attendants, beauticians were expected to provide service with a smile, yet they resisted internalizing these feelings. Instead, like other wage workers, beauty operators often relied on jokes and slang to articulate their own vision of the beauty process and one that was much less refined than what trade journals or beauty schools tried to project. Betty Saunders, who worked as an operator during the Depression, described how shop talk reinforced a collective identity that helped operators handle the daily stresses and strains in a manner that did not jeopardize their profit-making potential. A customer may ask for a facial massage, Saunders explained, but operators referred to the same treatment as giving their customers a "beating," while skin creams, finger waves, and henna rinse were described in less refined fashion as "hamburger," a "Hitch-Hike," and a "fire drill," respectively. A "set of whiskers" humorously described a woman wearing artificial eyelashes and a "harvest" meant a customer was having her eyebrows plucked. "Plastered," Saunders continued, simply meant the customer's "hair [was] set with special goo." There were also nicknames for customers. A "sponge," was generally "a good customer because she soaks up all the treatment." And although some beauticians may have shared their slang with a few favorite patrons, it was less likely that they did so when dealing with a "heavyweight" (or "high class customer"), a "schreech" (better known as a "complaining woman"), or a disappointing "Santa Claus" who only came to the shop "once a year."[57]

Operators also had to deal with an assortment of new hair products that were equally temperamental. Beauty shop mishaps were so common that advice columns became a regular feature in many trade journals. For example, in each issue of *The American Hairdresser*, Madam Louise's "Trouble Corner" answered questions dealing with everything from which shampoos were best to how to handle severe skin diseases. One of the most common complaints stemmed from unexpected changes in hair color: "Will you please let me know what can be done to blonde hair that has turned green after a permanent?" wrote one perplexed reader.

I have been doing this kind of work for five years and this lady had been my client ever since. The hair is just green in places near the roots of the hair. The only bleach used was peroxide-ammonia and, one other time, white henna. I have given her waves other times and they came out fine. What can I do to remove the color? At first it was brown—now it is green.[58]

Sometimes desperation even drove readers to send in samples of damaged hair for diagnosis.

> Could you explain the trouble which I am having with the hair I am enclosing? The bit of hair that is not in cellophane is hair to which I gave a permanent wave. I steamed it four and one-half minutes, using _____ solution. When it was taken from the rods it was very curly but as it was wetted it became more limp. After a month, it was perfectly straight. the hair in the cellophane paper is of the same head. I gave this lady another permanent wave on April 16, steamed four minutes using _____ solution.[59]

The new hair products with which operators had to deal also contributed to a variety of health risks that were just beginning to be investigated in the 1930s. Operators commonly suffered from "Beautician's Eczema," because they were "continually exposed to various chemicals" in "soaps, hair dyes, creams, astringents, oils, mud packs, shampoos, acids, perfumes, deodorants, antiseptics, etc." Dermatologist Morris M. Estrin was not surprised to find beauticians who "break out on the skin, especially the fingers, hands, wrists and arms, and even to the entire body which is especially dangerous." Estrin found injured skin that eventually became infected, particularly problematic. "Tiny blisters," he found, led to severe itching, and "ringworm infections" tended to spread from persistent scratching. Moreover, these infections were difficult to cure. "The skin between the fingers and the webs of the fingers are very tender, and once the eczema or ringworm gets a foot hold there, it usually takes many months" to cure. Nor were rubber gloves much help. Excluding washing and dyeing, gloves were a nuisance because they made many procedures difficult to perform. And *The American Hairdresser* warned that if rubber gloves were worn consistently, "the patron will become suspicious" and question the safety of the products being used on their own hair and skin.[60]

74   Headaches and sore throats were also a common complaint, especially among African-American operators. In a 1939 investigation of African-American beauty shops, investigators found that beauty operators frequently suffered from throat infections and headaches. Many beauty shops were located in basements that had little or no ventilation. "Operators or booth renters who remain in these places for long made complaints of 'having a headache all the time.'" Investigators warned that the "pressing of hair gives off carbon particles," which were inhaled by "operators [who] must stand over and very close to the hair that is being pressed." These fumes also irritated beauty operators' throats, and "if the hair is not washed immediately before pressing there is a great danger of infection." To help solve the problem, owners and operators often insisted that customers have their hair shampooed before they received any other services or, at the very least, they urged their customers to wash their hair at home before coming to the shop. In fact, operators would often charge the same price whether the hair was shampooed or not in order to encourage customers to have their hair washed before having it pressed.[61]

Beauticians suffered other aches and pains from handling cumbersome equipment. Alata Hogue, who owned a shop in Pomona, California, advised beauty operators to wear "An ordinary pair of canvas gardening gloves" when "handling the permanent wave machine." The gloves made it easier for operators "to reach the heaters quickly and to get in and out among them should the patron complain of too much heat in any spot." This was especially useful when "removing heaters rapidly after the steaming time is up." Hogue insisted that they saved her hands from the "many scars" usually found "on the operator's hands." Beauticians also complained of symptoms that in later decades would come to be defined as carpal tunnel syndrome. "The operator who gives many marcels often has trouble with her wrist," explained Madelyn Mae Montgomery, a beauty shop owner in Glendale, California. "I have found that it helps greatly to wear a wrist band while marcelling. You may get these bands in chamois or leather at any drug store." Montgomery also encouraged the operator to keep "the patron's chair low enough so that you can work with your elbows down. This is great saving of arm sockets."[62]

Beauticians also complained about the long hours of constantly standing on their feet, which was considered to be the trade's most detrimental aspect. According to the New York Labor Advisory Board, "the greatest objection to beauty shop work, from the point of view of the health and well-being of the employee, is the shockingly long hours" and the "constant standing."[63] Long hours were particularly problematic before holidays and towards the end of the work week, and it was a common practice in many shops to hire "week-end extras," many of whom were women still enrolled in beauty-culture courses. During rush periods, white, female operators typically worked from nine o'clock in the morning until nine o'clock at night. The busiest hours were from eleven o'clock until two o'clock, making lunch nothing more than a quick sandwich and a cold drink. More than one-fourth of the Euro-American women surveyed by the Advisory Board worked over forty-eight hours, and one in five worked at least ten hours a day. To be sure, in residential districts there was a great lack of uniformity in the hours of operation among different shops, but there were two characteristics that were fairly general in these neighborhood beauty parlors: long hours and evening work. In Manhattan, the neighborhood shop tended to open later in the morning than those in the central business district, but they also stayed open late into the evening. Three-fifths of the shops in residential neighborhoods were open until eight or later, while nearly half were open until nine or ten in the evening.[64]

African-American women's work days tended to be even longer and more irregular than those of their Euro-American counterparts. This primarily reflected the long hours associated with domestic workers, who made up the bulk of their beauty shop clientele. Thursdays were a particularly busy day for most operators since it was traditionally the domestic workers' day off. In the 1930s, Lydia Adams opened her first shop in Chicago on Forty-seventh and Michigan. "In the beginning many of our customers were working for white families doing private family work. They were making five to seven dollars a week [and] they had maybe Thursdays off and half day off [on] Sunday." Adams recalled how "they always had a dollar or a dollar and a half to get their hair done" and that was how she got "started."[65] Women's Bureau agents also discovered that Saturdays were busy for

African-American beauticians because it was the factory worker's pay day. In general, African-American operators faced closing times on Thursdays as late as nine or ten in the evening, sometimes as late as midnight, while Saturday appointments could stretch into the early hours of the morning.[66]

Seasonal fluctuations compounded the problems associated with irregular hours. In New York, investigators found that there were few shops whose business was "steady throughout the year." The busiest time of year was the spring, "especially during the permanent waving season from April to June." Investigations found that nearly half of all New York City's beauty parlors "make a practice of varying the size of their staffs with the volume of their business." While some businesses "take on extra workers for the busy season, some lay off their regular workers in the summers, and some do both." Summer "lay-offs" and/or "vacations without pay" were a common experience for the urban beautician. In places like Brooklyn and Queens, half of all operators found themselves unemployed during the summer. Occasionally they could find work at resorts or on ships, but most had to find work in other fields. And if a shop did not reduce the number of employees during the slack season, they would drop their hours or reduce their wages.[67]

To a large degree, seasonal fluctuations and summer layoffs reflected the fact that most beauty shops were not air conditioned and customers simply could not tolerate the heat. In the summer, shops were often hot and stuffy, and the use of permanent-wave machines and dryers made conditions unbearable. According to Helen Milner, an owner of a thirteen-booth shop in Cleveland, women were encouraged during the hot summer months "to have only absolutely necessary work done, and then get out into the open air as quickly as possible."[68] It was quite common during the hot weather to find customer traffic "slow up" and "listen to the complaints of 'It's so hot I can't stand having my hair dried' and similar remarks." The permanent wave in particular "looms so large in the patron's mind in connection with what she terms 'that awful heat.'" In response, some shops installed a "cooling system."[69] The Edythe Beauty Salon, located in St. Louis, Missouri, at Broadway and Chippewa in 1938, boasted the look and feel of modernity. Neon lights, "shaped like drawn drapes, of dark and light green, frame the large plate glass window." In the center of the window was the name of the shop and just below it "blue neon outlines [of] a beautifully coiffered head." Inside, the walls were orchid with "furniture of yellow leather and chrome." But it was "the new Chrysler Air Temp" that caught the attention of the casual passerby and made "even a summer permanent a pleasure."[70]

Of course air-conditioning was a luxury that only the larger more exclusive shops could afford, compelling other shop owners to search out less expensive methods to keep their clientele cool and comfortable. In St. Louis, Mrs. Clark's Hiawatha Beauty Salon, located just across the street from The Edythe Beauty Shop, occupied "a floor below the surface" where "a natural coolness prevails, making the shop inviting long before air-conditioning."[71] When Ida Connolly found that her customers suffered from the heat, the "only thing" she could do "to cool off the shop was to put a big wash tub in the center of the floor and have ice delivered twice a day." Connolly recalled that on some of those hot days "the customers and others would duck their hands up to their elbows in this ice water to cool themselves off." While the big tub of ice "helped a great deal," she still found that the heat generated from "the permanent wave machine and driers going" made doing business on hot summer days "next to impossible."[72] At the very least, *The American Hairdresser* insisted that "the best ventilation of the shop should be given to the room where this is conducted." Other "hot weather hints" included making "arrangements with a neighboring store" that was willing to serve cold drinks such as "lemonade, iced tea, or just cold water" or to install a "water cooler or mechanical refrigerator." All of these suggestions, *The American Hairdresser* believed, would help make customers more content and employees more efficient.[73]

While the heat bothered the clientele, it was the combination of low wages and long hours that operators found most unbearable. "Probably no group of workers in our state [Ohio] endures a greater burden in the way of oppressive and unreasonably low wages or resents this condition more bitterly than those engaged in beauty culture," insisted Dolly Phillips Hanline, a local union secretary in Akron.[74] During the Depression, the New York Department of Labor received similar complaints about long hours in beauty shops. New York shops, declared one beautician, request "an experienced operator who is expected to know everything from shampooing hair to permanent waving and hair dyeing," yet "the average salary" for most operators was about twelve dollars for working twelve hour days. Shops owners were also notorious for quoting "a certain salary to an employment agency in order to get an operator, and then ask you to work for about $5.00 less after the first week or two, which is most unjust to the operator, [and] inasmuch as 10 per cent of the first month's salary goes to the employment agency." It seemed unfair, another beautician protested, that "the average beauty parlor owner expects an operator to work for a starvation wage and depend on tips to make up for the scanty wages that he offers."[75]

The beautician's starvation wages did not go unnoticed, at least not by their customers. In June 1936, one customer complained to the New York Department of Labor of conditions in a shop she frequented, which she described as "appalling." "The girls work from twelve to fourteen hours a day; some girls receiving only 4 and 5 dollars a week." In her letter she asked if "there isn't some way of helping these girls? Can't you make it your business to see that they get shorter hours and higher wages?" A concerned shop owner in Buffalo, New York, insisted that the only way "cheap shops" managed to stay afloat was by exploiting their employees. Many shops, she insisted, were "turning out Permanent Waves [for] 75 cents, finger waves [at] 15 cents . . . [and] People wonder how they do this . . . they only pay them either a salary of $4.00 to $6.00," she protested, and "some of them a straight commission." Because of the low wages, some operators quit right after they started working, realizing it was impossible to make ends meet on such meager wages. In Buffalo, for example, one operator left her shop the very first day of work because she only made about 30 cents—"her carfare was 20 cents a day and then she had to buy her lunch—so you can imagine how much she would make if she stayed on." In other shops, this same Buffalo resident complained, the conditions were not only "deplorable," or so she had heard, but "a terrible fire-trap." Indeed, she was "surprised [that] a city like Buffalo would allow such a place to exist," although she admitted that when times are tough, "many people are attracted by cheap prices." At the same time, she felt "any one who had any respect for themselves won't go back."[76]

New York's public relief records also indicated problems in the beauty shop industry. The New York State Department of Labor along with the New York City Emergency Relief Bureau found beauty parlor employees "whose earnings were so low that they had to be supplemented from the public relief funds." In 1936, a number of women employed in beauty shops were receiving assistance from the city of New York. The Department of Labor's files, in particular, brought into question beauty shop wages. Sarah M., for example, was "an all-around operator earning $4.00, including tips for a 47 1/2 hour week in a Harlem Beauty Shop," which meant her hourly wage was only 8.4 cents. Mildred De M. earned twelve cents an hour as a manicurist. Her employer paid her two dollars for thirty-six hours of work each week, and she received an additional two dollars and thirty-five cents in tips. Another manicurist, described in the Labor department's file as "a deserted Negress supporting two others," earned 16.7 cents an hour or four dollars a week for twenty-four hours worth of work.[77]

Low wages and long hours also meant beauty shops faced an unusually high turnover rate, suggesting that employees often resisted with their feet. In 1933, Marian Varley of New York City complained that during the two years she had been in business, she "must have been employed in about twenty five different shops." Much to her dismay, they all offered "cut rate prices," ranging anywhere from twenty to thirty-five cents. Moreover, it seemed that these cut-rate shops were the "only positions available in any employment agency."[78] Indeed, several employment agencies in New York City found that while some shops kept a small proportion of their employees for up to twelve months, many operators changed jobs "twice or even three or four times a year." In fact, a survey done by Bryn Mawr summer school students indicated that the turnover rate in the mid-1920s was higher for beauticians than for female industrial workers: "over three-quarters of these [industrial] workers had held their jobs on an average of a year or longer and more than two-fifths, on an average of two or more years," while beauty parlors were either going out of business or others were opening up, contributing "to the instability of employment in this field."[79]

Differences in wages also tended to fall along lines of race and gender. While Euro-American and African-American women generally worked as "all-around operators," there were dramatic differences in their earnings. In 1934, the Women's Bureau found that in four cities—Philadelphia, New Orleans, St. Louis, and Columbus, Ohio—a quarter of all Euro-American women and two-thirds of all African-American women surveyed earned less than ten dollars a week. The average weekly wage ranged from a little over fourteen dollars for Euro-American women to as little as eight dollars for African-American operators. And tips generally amounted to no more than one or two dollars more each week. In contrast, a disproportionate number of white men worked as specialists and were often hired only to do bobbing, permanent waving, marcelling, or dyeing. Their average salary was twenty-two dollars and fifty cents.[80] In New York, investigators found that "every shop of any size employs at least one man and some of the large shops have as many as 50 men." White men were disproportionately located in the most exclusive salons where they enjoyed "shorter [hours] and less irregular" work than their female counterparts.[81]

Men also boasted that they were more competent than the typical beautician. In 1927, *The Journeyman Barber* published an article that insisted that success in the beauty business depended upon a "competent man barber to do the work, as the customers will no longer have an inexperienced girl butcher up their hair." Indeed, "the reason barbershops became popular in the first place," the article claimed, was because of "the disappointment women experienced when they went to a beauty parlor and the work was done by a girl."[82]

Of course gender differences diminished once race was taken into account. One of the ways beauticians challenged the poor conditions in which they worked was to organize, and often with the encouragement of barbers. By the early twentieth century, white and black journeyman barber locals had been organized across the country. The disproportionate numbers of African-American barbers compelled white-dominated unions to recognize some black workers, and, above the Mason-Dixon line, African-American barbers organized separately. The one exception or group excluded were Asians. Women were welcomed, according to James C. Shanessy, General President of the Journeyman Barbers, who "called the memberships' attention" to the need to organize beauticians and hairdressers. In fact, Shanessy directed union membership to the constitution, which clearly explained that "Any competent journeyman barber, hairdresser, waver, marceller or cosmetician other than a member of an Oriental race" was welcome to join the Journeymen.[83]

Although there had been some longstanding tension between barbers and hairdressers, each fearing each other's encroachment on the trade, barbers cast the need to organize women not in terms of competition but rather benevolence. Barbers described beauticians as victims of "starvation wages" and unbearably long hours.[84] According to Shanessy, beauty parlors were kept "open until all hours of the night and work their assistants inhumanely for long hours for a small wage and still smaller commission; in all barely making a living." And if beauticians were not organized, barbers feared that they would "pay a tremendous price for it" because beauticians were after all "in competition with the average barbershop."[85]

Unfortunately for barbers, beauticians were not always so anxious to organize with men and even expressed a certain amount of ambivalence. When a Bronx local joined efforts with the Women's Trade Union League (WTUL), they found "the response of the girls to the organization was very slow." Not because they "were entirely indifferent to organization," explained Sadie Reisch of the WTUL, "but there was sort of a superior air about them." Indeed, she claimed that "the beauty parlor workers looked down upon the barbers and at the beginning of the strike the girls absolutely refused to join the same local with the barbers." According to Reisch, even after a strike was called, the "girls" initially "refused to be out picketing or to be active in any way." Instead, Reisch complained that "they thought that everything ought to be handed to them on a silver platter." Yet their ambivalence was not simply because of "a superior air." One beautician who worked at an "unusually neat and up-to-date beauty shop" simply stated that she "was not going to have the union telling me what to do." Beauticians not only feared that the union would try to dictate prices, hours, and the conditions under which thy were expected to work, but that the male-dominated journeyman barber union wanted to "control the beautician."[86]

Barbers and beauticians did mount a number of successful

unionization drives in cities across the country.[87] But bonds between beauticians and customers proved to be more enduring than those between beautician and barber. Indeed, unionization never seemed as pervasive or successful for beauticians who worked in small owner-operated shops. Instead, the relationships beauticians developed with their customers were relied upon to counter workplace demands. In 1929, Philadelphia shop owner Joseph De Silvis insisted that "our greatest problem" in the industry was not unions, but "the operator who makes a few special customers and then tries to hold the proprietor up for more money and special considerations." De Silvis, who employed "forty to fifty operators in three of the largest beauty parlors in Philadelphia," declared that he would "no longer tolerate clients who count on one special operator for their work." "Nothing," he insisted, "disrupts an organization more quickly than allowing operators to become intimate with the customer." De Silvis tried to reason with his customers by taking them into his "confidence" and "to make them realize the evil effect such practice has on the moral of the rest." But he found the loyalty between customer and operator too difficult to break, compelling him to resort to what he called "another good remedy for this evil." Undoubtedly influenced by methods of scientific management, De Silvis broke down the work process, and instead of hiring all-around beauticians, he had his "operators specialize in certain branches of beauty work" to ensure that there were "no favorite customers or favored operators" and that "one operator will not be in a position to monopolize the customers by creating the impression that they know it all." De Silvis boasted that his operators were "schooled to give the best work impersonally" and urged other shop owners to do the same if they wanted to solve "This Help Problem."[88]

Unlike De Silvis, most shop owners could not afford to hire enough beauty operators for each individual task, but *The American Hairdresser* thought that shop owners could keep operators' conversations from becoming too personal. Shop rules, one editorial insisted, "should warn against loud, animated conversation from one booth to another." *The American Hairdresser* also felt that it was not "good form" for "some operators [to] call their customers 'Honey,' or 'Dear,'" which was sometimes common "after the second meeting" and specifically forbade any "discussion as to preference in colors for costumes, criticism or detailing of another customer's affairs or habits, [like] the dance attended last night."[89] Susan Porter Benson argues that saleswomen used such conversations as a way to defy their subordinate position behind the counter.[90] Beauty operators relied on the familiarity bred by conversation in a similar fashion, and while it mitigated class differences between operator and client, it also created gendered alliances between worker and customer. *The American Hairdresser* warned shop owners that gossip between hairdressers and beauty shop patrons was not merely a question of propriety, but a direct challenge to managerial control. Hazel Koslay, editor-in-chief of *The American Hairdresser*, asked her readership, "Who Owns Your Shop . . . You or Your Operators?" "Far too often" Koslay found that beauty parlors were "in the grip of the employees." Indeed, "the older the salon, the more serious is the situation," especially "in those shops where the operators have been allowed to build up a close following." Shop owners, Koslay explained, feared that disgruntled employees "will move on to another shop and take their customers with them." And "there is always the threat, too, of the operator leaving to open her own place of business with a substantial and ready-made following whose loss to you will have serious consequences."[91]

"Prevention," Hazel Koslay insisted, was "so much easier than [a] cure, in a situation of this sort." "The best and old-established shop," she thought, should "slowly wean customers away from operators, either by having another operator serve them occasionally, or by the owner herself taking over, when it can be done diplomatically on, for instance, a very busy day of the operator whose association seems too close." She also argued that newer shops should never allow customers to become emotionally attached to the operators. "Keep your own personal contacts with customers close enough," she explained, "so they feel they depend on you and the salon for service they like, and not on any one operator." At the least, Koslay cautioned shop owners to enter into the service in an "advisory capacity," and they should "change customers from one operator to another, tactfully, as much as you can . . . always injecting your own personality and value into the picture."[92]

Shop owners were particularly uncomfortable with the practice of beauticians taking their clientele elsewhere, prompting an anonymous New York owner to suggest a systematic method of blacklisting that would punish "unscrupulous employees" as well as conspiring shop owners. In a letter to the New York Hairdressers and Cosmetologists Association, this owner complained about beauty operators who for "some reason" become "disgruntled with their employer" and "decide to change their place of employment." But before they leave, "these employees make a habit of getting the names and addresses of as many of the shop's customers as they can." They then have the audacity to "go to a competitive shop in the neighborhood and ask for a position, saying that they have a following." Of course, the other shop, "wanting to increase its business will employ the operator" who will be sure to "let the customers know her new place of employment." All in all, the shop owner described it as "a vicious practice which hurts the shop and gives the operator an unfair advantage over the employer." Also, it seemed that "new operators not from a competitive shop, do not bring any following," and thus the shop owner insisted that "it is wrong that they take anybody away." As a result, this writer suggested "that those owners who make it a practice of advertising for help with a following, or employ operators who state that they have such following, from competitive shops in the neighborhood, be warned to discontinue such practice." If they continued the practice, he argued, they should "be expelled from the association" and "Employees, who take the names and addresses of patrons should be discharged and be put on a blacklist."[93]

Thus the seemingly trivial conversations that came to characterize the everyday operations of the beauty shop not only provided beauticians with one of the most effective means to negotiate labor issues, but also held out the possibility of entrepreneurship and the kind of independence few service workers enjoyed. Beauty operators were well aware that there was little chance of advancement within shops and thus many beauticians attempted to move to better locations or open their own businesses. Within large shops, in particular, there tended to be a rigid hierarchy, and "The girl employed as a general operator in a beauty parlor in New York City had little chance for advancement in rank within the shop." If an operator was unusually talented in something such as permanent waving or dyeing, she might be hired as a specialist and enjoy higher wages and more regular hours. But since the majority of shops were small and employed primarily general operators and manicurists, chances for advancement were even less common. Only on occasion did investigators find manicurists who picked up other skills and became all-around operators. Usually, women either owned or managed a beauty shop or advanced their position in a shop by developing a loyal following that provided them the leverage they needed to negotiate a more favorable work environment.[94]

Lucille Miller felt that her fifteen years of hairdressing in Cleveland, Ohio made her judgment of the industry "fair" and "reliable." Through the first few decades of the twentieth century, the hairdressing industry was plagued with contradictions. Beauty schools frequently advertised beauty culture and hairdressing as a way to earn a decent living and enjoy an occupation surrounded with glamour, style, and independence. Yet operators were often disillusioned and found that once they completed their schooling, they had to struggle against starvation wages and ten- to twelve-hour work days. Moreover, the conditions in which beauty operators worked were often unbearable. The occupational hazards ranged from chemical burns to ill-ventilated shops. All this seemed to fly in the face of the investment some women made in training and education. As well, beauty operators often faced conflicting policies with managers who insisted that they cater to their clients' every need yet act "professional" and depersonalize their service. In response, beauticians not only moved from shop to shop until they found a more suitable work culture but also ignored managerial policies and relied heavily upon the operator-client relationship to negotiate workplace demands. To be sure, the relationships that formed between beauticians and their clients could be contentious. The ability to curry favor with customers relied on as much skill and imagination as some of the most elaborate coiffures. But the operator-customer relationship proved far too elusive for owners and managers to control. The intimacy that characterized shop culture and the hairdresser-client relationship along with the services operators had to offer during good times and bad usually led to bonds customers were unwilling to break, providing beauticians with the relationships they needed to create a more pleasing work culture.

Beauty operators' working conditions would only get worse before they improved, however. With the Depression and New Deal legislation, small-time entrepreneurs were no longer simply having to deal with long hours and low wages but would suddenly find themselves and their businesses blamed not only for increased competition but also for the industry's tarnished image. Beauticians' efforts to deal with the Depression and industry leaders' attempts to professionalize beauty culture constituted the greatest contradiction operators faced.

3

Blue Eagles, Neighborhood Shops, and the Making of a Profession

L aura Wernsman lived in Eureka, Illinois, during the Great Depression of the 1930s. She never had "any schooling in Barbering or Beauty Culture work," but according to Laura, what mattered most was that she knew how to style hair and had managed to develop a clientele composed of a few of her "poor friends and neighbors." One day in the fall of 1933, "a Chicago man with a V-8 Ford car came to [her] place." "He read us the law," remembered Laura, and, much to her dismay, he insisted that neither she nor her sister could "set or cut hair anymore." Her sister even had to "sign her name" on a piece of paper, promising "she would not wave or cut hair." But to Laura it seemed unlikely that this "Chicago man" could actually stop them from doing their neighbors' hair and more possible that he was a "fake." Laura's suspicions prompted her to memorize his Illinois license plate number and write to the National Recovery Administration (NRA) to find out whether or not his claims were legitimate and if it was really "against the law to cut or set hair, without charging or without having schooling or [a] license?"[1]

Like Laura Wernsman, hundreds of women working in the beauty industry wrote to the federal government for answers, advice, and help as they faced not only the "iron hands of the Depression," but also New Deal attempts to regulate the industry through the NRA, which threatened to undermine the livelihood of countless numbers of working women and small entrepreneurs. The push to regulate the industry emerged with the growth of "popularly-priced" beauty shops in the early 1920s. Before the Depression, various laws regarding the age and educational requirements of beauty operators affected men and women in just a few states, and there were no federal guidelines designed to restructure the industry until the first wave of New Deal legislation. Ultimately, the Depression created a crisis in hairdressing as it did in many industries, but this crisis also served as a golden opportunity for those who had long sought regulation. Although a national beauty code was never legally signed into law, associations composed of exclusive shop owners attempted to establish laws determining everything from who could work as a hairdresser and where a business could be located to when it could operate and how much could be charged, all of which would force many of the more modest shops to close their doors, ensuring a less competitive market. In theory, the NRA was designed to create "codes of fair competition" in each industry, healing the country from the downward spiral of "cut-throat and monopolistic price slashing." The NRA urged industries across the country to collectively submit a code of self-regulation, pledging to end child labor, pay a minimum wage of twelve to thirteen dollars per week, and maintain a maximum forty-hour work week. In return, each business could display the Blue Eagle as a symbol of compliance and civic responsibility.[2] Once regulation was intertwined with New Deal legislation and American patriotism, reform efforts found far more legitimacy than in previous years. Indeed, now rather than being described as an "amateur shop," the neighborhood beautician was a "cut-throat" competitor and a "chiseler" who threatened to undermine not only the beauty industry but also the nation's economic recovery.

In their letters to the federal government, beauty operators and small shop owners expressed ambivalence towards the establishment of an NRA code in the hairdressing industry. While beauty operators exhibited a strong desire to "do their part" for the recovery, they voiced concerns over the establishment of a code that threatened their work, identity, and economic well-being. Their letters reveal just how crucial the smallest shops were to the development of the industry and to the survival of thousands of families. Above all, they expose the contradictions between the goals of hairdressing associations and working-class women's daily survival strategies. According to hundreds of female entrepreneurs, the NRA favored top-down decision making and definitions of business legitimacy that jeopardized the vast majority of small neighborhood businesses. National hairdressing associations along with various state and local organizations were concerned with the image of the industry, which the unprecedented growth of "amateur" shops typically located in the kitchens, lavatories, and front rooms of flats and private homes had tarnished. The neighborhood shop, they argued, was a place where inexperience compromised both worker and consumer.

But concerns over exploitation and inexperience were only part of a larger agenda; regulation also would aid industry leaders' quest for professionalism and respectability. Professionalism, as understood by most contemporaries, was a male-defined, middle-class ideology, even though hairdressing was primarily a working-class female occupation. This inherent contradiction resulted in the attempt by national associations to redefine beauty culture in terms of a masculine, middle-class "white-collar" world of work and business. The NHCA, for example, did not consider the beauty shop a legitimate business unless it stood clearly beyond the boundaries of domestic space and traditional household chores. Nor would a woman have been considered a qualified hairdresser if she merely learned to style hair through the course of girlhood like Laura Wernsman. Education, instead, had to be formalized and standardized to the degree that even apprenticeship was deemed unacceptable.

As much as this quest for respectability stemmed from a gendered and class-based definition of professionalism, it was also an issue complicated by race. Hairdressing was a female occupation regardless of the industry's male leadership, yet it was also defined as a service industry. Beauticians were commonly classified with domestics, porters, maids, and other workers who were characterized as less respectable and less white. During the Depression, the line between the Euro-American beauty-culture industry and other non-white service work was blurred as the forms of exploitation experienced by beauticians were commonly expressed through racial metaphors. Young, white, female beauty operators, for example, were often described by the NHCA as victims of "sweat-shops" who worked like "slaves" at "coolie-level wages." Although the need to increase operators' pay to the level of a living wage seemed self-evident, leaders from Euro-American hairdressing associations argued for increases because beauty operators' weekly wages were uncomfortably close to those earned by African Americans and immigrant workers. To be sure, many of these same racial metaphors were used to describe other workers who faced poor wages and working conditions during the Depression, but the Euro-American hairdressing industry's quest for legitimacy and the historical significance of black women in the industry made issues of race more problematic. Ultimately, then, it was not simply professional aspirations but the dangerous closeness of beauty culture to service work and thus to people of color that was so problematic.

In 1934, the NHCA emerged as the leading sponsor of a NRA code for hairdressing, but their efforts to reform the industry began a decade earlier with the dramatic growth of popularly priced beauty shops. In 1921, the NHCA's First Annual Convention began to look at ways to uplift the industry's image and focused specifically on the issue of "itinerant workers," the need for a standardized hairdressing textbook and recognized schools, and other "ethical issues" to ensure fair business practices. By 1923, the NHCA's agenda focused on the "influx of permanent wave machine manufactures and the sale of home permanent waving 'outfits,'" which in their words had become a "growing problem." It seemed that "These machines were being sold to anyone, and many untrained persons were entering the field, causing cut prices."[3] Indeed, prices had plummeted well before the Depression. "Years ago [1910s] when Permanent waveing first came out," customers regularly paid as much as twenty-five dollars for their curls. In the 1920s, the price dropped to fifteen dollars, and, according to F. A. Hood of Margaret Hood's Beauty Salon, everyone "thought it was just terrible." But by the end of the decade, permanents had dropped to as low as two dollars, making a trip to the beauty shop affordable even for working-class women.[4]

There were also complaints from hairdressers across the country that beauty schools were by and large nothing more than "diploma mills" that flooded the market with poorly trained beauty operators.[5] The NHCA and other hairdressing associations found it necessary to rigidly distinguish the legitimate hairdresser who was both a businessman and a highly trained beauty specialist from working-class women who worked in their homes or, even worse, went door-to-door doing finger waves for as little as fifteen cents. The NHCA reported that the number of beauty operators tripled between 1920 and 1930, and nearly half of their membership agreed that their "greatest competitors were 'Bathroom beauty shops.'" Most disturbing from the NHCA's perspective was that these small "illegitimate" businesses proved to be the cornerstone of the beauty-culture industry.[6]

Echoing NHCA sentiment, the National Women's Trade Union League (WTUL) was also concerned that the beauty industry had grown uncontrollably and "literally by leaps and bounds." In their words, the beauty-culture industry had become "'big business' and a highly specialized profession," and one that now constituted "a nationwide industrial problem" that needed to be investigated. They estimated that the Chicago vicinity alone boasted as many as 4,500 beauty parlors, many of which were in the "'front room' in the residence, where the housewife sandwiches a shampoo in between household duties." This type of shop, the WTUL insisted, was "looked upon by the profession much as were the 'sweat shops' in the garment industry." And thus "the small home shop," they concluded, "may [soon] be weeded out in Illinois, due to a new state law and city zoning restrictions." "Not only must the public be safeguarded against health hazards," but the WTUL also noted that hours, wages, and working conditions needed to be improved for the sake of female employees.[7]

The Consumer's League of New York City provided an investigation of fifty-four beauty shops and confirmed the WTUL and the NHCA's assumptions that the industry was in desperate need of standardization. According to the WTUL, the investigation revealed all kinds of problems and proved that officials needed to decide exactly "who may do what" in the profession. Concerns continued to focus exclusively on "underbidding, amateur shops," especially those with "the owner living under the same roof" and which "have a way of springing up over night." The Consumer's League found that the "better shops are asking for the protection of patrons," and that the industry needed state laws to "establish cosmeticians' boards for the licensing of shops, the inspection of sanitary conditions and health hazards, and the qualifications and training of operators." The state of California served as a model because "the beauty parlor industry had been placed in the hands of a board of unpaid cosmetologists appointed by the Governor [which] made all kinds of standards" and placed "the whole industry upon a professional basis." A professional basis, however, translated into strict limitations designed to discourage apprenticeship and most significantly to "prohibit beauty operators from working in their apartments or homes."[8] "No longer should a wash bowl and turkish towel designate a 'beauty parlor,' and an old kitchen chair and apron and old shears, a barber shop."[9]

Regardless of the motive, proving to legislators that the hairdressing industry needed regulation in the name of consumer protection took little convincing. Stories of beauty shop mishaps and homemade disasters shaped the collective memory of a generation of women who came of age with the first permanent-wave machines and a vast array of hairstyling techniques, dyes, and solutions. For Billie Jones Kanan, disappointing results paled only in comparison to the suffering she endured from her first trip to the beauty shop. "It must have been about 1928 when my mother, my sister and I all got permanents in St. Joseph, [Missouri]," recalled Kanan. "It took all day, and cost $1 each," but that was not the worst of it. "As I recall, I couldn't have cared less about curls, but went along and was tortured beyond my wildest imagination." Kanan remembered every detail of the process. "First our hair was washed and cut, then we waited and waited. There were women everywhere in different stages of getting beautified. Everyone was waiting." Once the waiting ended, Kanan explained that the real torture began. "My hair was wound up on spiral rods so tight that I thought I would never blink again [and] after the machine that looked like a milking machine was attached to the rods, I couldn't move. [Then] it all began to steam and tears rolled down my cheeks." Finally, her suffering caught an operator's attention. "Someone got a blower and cooled my head here and there, but my scalp was scalded." Her mother thought she "should have said something sooner." But at the time, she assumed that "maybe this was just a part of being beautiful." That notion quickly vanished, however, when she looked in the mirror and found that the closest thing her blonde hair now resembled was a "haystack."[10] "Getting beautified" for Gwen Jeschke was equally devastating. As a young girl, she repeatedly suffered at the hands of an inexperienced operator. After her first permanent wave she did everything she could "to keep from screaming." "It was awful," she remembered, because "it stuck out all over the place." Jeschke, however, did not learn from her initial mistake. "When this permanent grew out," she confessed that she tried it again and once again "something" went "wrong, because it was really fluffy." She was embarrassed when her "girl friend saw it." But there was no way to hide it. "How could she miss it! It looked like I'd stuck my finger in a light socket."[11]

Even women who were pleased with the end results never forgot suffering from cumbersome equipment and an occasional burn. At the age of "12 or 13 years old, having curly hair was one of my most important wishes," remembered Flora Pyles, a woman from Union Star, Missouri. Every spring her mother and four of her friends would take an annual trip to Maysville "to get permanents." Finally, after she "begged and pleaded," her parents "consented for [her] to have curly hair." "The five of us left home early in the morning to go to Miss Brant's Beauty Shop in Maysville as an entire day was needed to get the new look." The cost of a cut and a permanent was usually one dollar, but this particular operator occasionally "ran a special for 89 cents." Pyles recalled the process in detail. "First came the haircut, and then she rolled the hair on the rods. Each rod was enclosed in a heavy clamp-like device which was attached by electric cords to a stand above your head [that] heated the rolled hair until the desired curl developed." Pyles remembered that "it was a long ordeal" and "sometimes you got scalp burns and the weight on your head was so heavy that if you leaned one way or the other, it was hard to straighten up your head." But she seemed satisfied with her new look. "When the process was over you could really be sure of tight curls," and although "a few didn't turn out well," admitted Pyles, "most did."[12]

Even beauty operators confessed that they were guilty of disastrous mistakes. African-American women were especially prone to burns from a hot comb or curling iron that was typically heated on a stove or in a fire and used to press hair straight or into smooth waves. Kathyrn Gamble, who grew up in "a family of eight girls, all with long, thick hair," visited the beauty shop only on occasion. As children, their "hair was washed in the beautiful soft rainwater and braided tight," but as they "grew older, [they] learned to use the hot comb." By the time Gamble entered high school, she "had been to the beauty shop often enough to learn how to use curling irons." "I would watch the hairdresser's hands," she insisted, "then go home and practice on my sisters." "Before long I was doing a pretty good job on friends and neighbors." That is until one day when she was working on one of her regular customers, an "elderly woman and a good neighbor, Aunt Hattie." Things were going well, but just as Gamble finished what she "thought was a good job," Aunt Hattie suddenly became upset. "She didn't say a word but started hitting me with a towel" and it was at that the moment Gamble realized that "The comb must have been a little too hot for her." "She scared me to death," remembered Gamble, who "ran all the way home [and] never went back to fix Aunt Hattie's hair."[13]

By the early years of the Depression, beauty operators frequently complained about worn out equipment and supplies, increasing the potential for disaster and health risks. Marian Varley worked as a manicurist, "finger waver," and all-around operator in New York City. In just two years, she had worked in twenty-five different shops, all of which she described as "cut-throat sweat shops" where the prices for various services ranged from twenty to thirty-five cents. Varley reported one Bronx beauty shop to the board of health that habitually used "dirty towels for facials," but the problem seemed unsolvable because "most every one of these cut rate shops use soiled towels." Her worst experience was in a shop located in the neighborhood of St. Nicholas Avenue and 178th Street where she was hired to do finger waving and manicures. "During the two months I was there, I must have worked any where from ten to twelve hours overtime every week

without receiving any extra pay." After the owner discovered she
was also trained to do permanent waving, the owner expected
Varley to help her when she became too busy to complete a permanent. Typically, one operator would begin to process a permanent wave, and another would finish. One day, "I had finished
winding a customers hair," she explained, "and was told to take a
lunch break, [while] the other operator did the baking." After
lunch, Varley "discovered the customer had a scalp burn." A
quick inspection of the equipment revealed that the shop owner
had carelessly "used her pads so many times they had holes in
them." Despite repeated warnings, the owner "disregarded [Var-
ley's] advice to get rid of them." While Varley was soon fired, she
took satisfaction in learning that "one of her customers sued [the
owner] for one thousand dollars."[14]

During the depths of the Depression, shop owners found that
they simply could not afford to replace equipment despite consumer risks. Several beauty operators in Burlington, Iowa insisted
that each one of their shops "has from two to five thousand dollars worth of machinery and equipment in it." But because of constant use over a four to five year period, the equipment was "practically worn out." In 1934, a new hair dryer cost at least one hundred dollars, while a new permanent wave machine cost three
hundred dollars. "Every shop is badly in need of new electrical
equipment," and "the public is in danger when shops are being
forced to use old worn out electrical equipment badly in need of
repair." The Burlington operators declared that unless the NRA
hairdressing code was approved, which would force an increase
in prices, they would not be "able to still keep up [their] former
standard of clean, safe, sanitary conditions," nor would they be
in a position to "give the public the time and care which should
be given them when giving a permanent wave," all of which they
warned could lead to "some of the most horrible accidents ever
known." Many of these accidents, argued the Burlington operators, were already "happening every day." And "by all means"
they felt that "the public must be protected from the under-cut-
ting, chiseling shop owner" who does not think about the
"human lives that are entrusted to their care."[15]

The NHCA estimated that there were "on average three
[injuries] per shop per year" and thus a minimum of 168,000

accidents. Mr. George Mause represented the NHCA and testified before the NRA on the frequency and severity of "casualties sustained" in beauty parlors. While Mause noted that he could only estimate the frequency of injuries, he "found some shops admitting to as many as one injury a week." One of the most common complaints were the burns from chemical solutions, permanent-wave machines, hot irons, and driers. Finger waving could also lead to scalp burns, which on occasion became infected and resulted in "considerable pain and suffering by the injured" as well as "visits to the doctor" and "surgical operations." Even manicuring could cause serious infections that could "extend into the marrow [of the] bone, requiring severe surgical operations" and even the loss of fingers, arms, and "sometimes the loss of life." As well, it seemed that all kinds of injuries occurred in connection "with arching the eyebrows, bleaching of hair, dyeing of hair, . . . Marcel irons, hair driers, [and] inflammable shampoos."[16] Rather than blame hard times, the NHCA believed "as the profession grew, many unqualified practitioners, suppliers and manufacturers had entered the field and the profession," causing the dramatic increase in beauty-shop mishaps. Because the NHCA ignored the African-American beauty-culture industry, most complaints centered on white-owned shops of modest means and the problems associated with permanent-wave machines. One tragedy "receiving wide publicity" told the story of a woman "under a permanent wave machine [who] fainted." As the story goes, "the hairdresser, to revive her, threw water in her face and she was electrocuted." There were other sensational stories in the media about poison lipstick, while hair dyes were notorious for causing injuries and even death.[17] "[W]ithout any doubt," Mause declared, beauty shop patrons had become the victims of the "cheapest material."[18]

According to the NHCA, the cheapest material was used primarily in the small shops located in working-class communities. Mrs. Esther Johnson, vice president of the Chicago Hairdressers Association, a branch of the NHCA, owned a large shop that employed twenty operators. She believed small shop owners were fooling consumers into thinking that they were receiving a "genuine" product when they entered the neighborhood shop. In regard to lotions being used in setting the hair, beauty operators were not as "qualified as chemists," she declared, and should never "mix and prepare their own solutions." "Yet the unsuspecting patron allows any and all kinds of solutions to be used on her hair, without question, only for the reason that she has confidence in the shop she is in, and that because the shop owners says 'We make our own' it is safe." The NHCA insisted that "home shops" were owned and operated "by women who have never seen a beauty school," making them the greatest threat to the consumer.[19]

Many hairdressers also blamed the neighborhood shop for poor working conditions and low wages. Describing herself as "just another operator," Daisy Schwartz sought to expose the inner workings of New York's beauty shops or what she called "sweat shops." In a letter addressed to Eleanor Roosevelt, Schwartz asked if something could be "done to remedy this condition?" It was not merely for herself that she asked for Roosevelt's help, "but for 18 thousand operators in New York besides the many more in other states who are also having trouble." "Cut-rate shops" attract their customers by offering "three items for one dollar, and in that way they manage to keep going, by paying their operators the sum of five and six dollars a week salary and working them 12 and 14 hours a day," and, of course "still they fly the N.R.A. Banner." "It stands to reason that there are certain classes of people who can not afford to pay very much to have finger waves shampoo's or manicure's," Schwartz admitted, "but it seems to me that they could manage to pay fifty cents in an upstairs shop so that the Bosses might be able to pay a living wage to the operators." Schwartz also argued that prices must be increased because "a girl can not live on five dollars a week in New York." "We need more than anything the help of the public," she explained. "To let them know the things they are also up against, [such as unsanitary conditions] when they enter a cut rate shop."[20]

Most beauty operators also found themselves facing a factory-like mentality. Nathaniel Colby, President of the League of Master Beauticians, believed that "the depressed wages . . . bring conditions for most of us down to almost coolie level," and "the inhumanly long hours and meager pay envelopes of ninety per cent of all engaged in the industry, are truly tragic."[21] Besides poor wages, the New York Department of

Labor found that beauty operators were working constantly on their feet from twelve to fourteen hours a day and were barely able to "snatch a sandwich 'between customers.'" "Long hours in beauty shops having become a tradition," asserted the Labor Advisory Board, "owing in part to the fact that beauty shop employees have not been covered by labor laws in many states, since the majority of such laws were passed before women worked in large number in beauty parlors and before the public had become aware of existing abuses." Neighborhood shops catering to a working-class clientele were particularly problematic. In order to serve "business women who are at work during the day," the "custom" in some shops was to stay open "until 11 and 12 o'clock at night." In contrast, "the owner of the better type of establishment" had long believed that "long hours for his employees were unnecessary and objectionable."[22]

Of course, while New York's "upstairs" beauty shops were notorious for their poor working conditions, some of Chicago's more reputable department stores were arguably just as exploitative. "My dear President," wrote Jean Gray,

> I believe that your ears are never closed to the call of those who are suffering under the iron hands of depression and injustice. . . . I am one of the many thousands of women, in the city of Chicago who are beauty operators, and who have been exploited and taken advantage of to the extent that many of my sisters have been driven into the streets to sell their bodies to gain sufficient income upon which to live.

Gray was thankful, however, for she was one of the lucky ones— her husband earned eighteen dollars a week. "Out of what little we have I have been helping girl operators who did not have money to buy food and who are working with me in the beauty shop of the Davis Department store." Gray went on to complain about the department store where "we operators are paid a fifty percent commission on work done regardless of the fact that the Davis Dept. store is operating under the N.R.A." As an "experienced operator," Gray earned six to eight dollars a week, and this, she insisted, was the case "in the majority of the beauty parlors in and out of the department stores in this city." "Some months ago," she had written to the Chicago branch of the N.R.A. outlining the conditions she and other operators faced. "Now my dear President I am praying to whatever God there may be, that this letter comes to your eyes and that out of your great heart may come some way to help these forgotten women in their dire need."[23]

Despite the fact that the department-store beauty parlor seemed as problematic as any other shop, the small neighborhood shop was singled out as the greatest threat to the well-being of customers, beauty operators, and even well-established businesses. By 1933, Mrs. J. H. Riggan, a member of the Texas Association of Accredited Beauty Culturists, Inc., had "served in this profession for forty years," yet she had "never known conditions to be so as they are now." During the past two years, she found that "there have been many outsiders who have entered our profession and cut legitimate prices," and "many of our best shops have closed their doors." Shop owners' problems were made worse, Riggan complained, by the increasing numbers of "girls" who began "leaving legitimate shops, taking their clientele from the shops where they were previously employed, to do work in the customer's home." "Now, unless a code of fair competitive prices is established," she warned, "we will be in a worse condition than we are now, as the bottleggers of our profession, the price cutters and house to house operators, and the home shop with little or no investment, will continue to work havoc in our profession."[24]

Shop owners in other parts of the country agreed that the profession needed to rid itself of amateurs. Mrs. Carol B. Hepburn owned what she described as a "first class shop" in Hammonton, New Jersey, but found that she could no longer "compete with girls who fingerwave in lavatories and dressing rooms in several factories for 25 c" or with "a woman washing heads in her bathroom and [doing] fingerwaves in an upstairs bedroom for 25 c an item."[25] Miss Hazel Bartholf, who owned the Blue Bird Beauty Shop and who lived in a "small community of about 2800," thought that "women should be prohibited from using their kitchen sinks, bath rooms, [and] living rooms." The NRA, she hoped, would "do away with working in the homes" or "going from house to house." "There are too many operating over the country in this manner, and it is a detriment to the profession."[26]

Shop owners also argued that kitchen beauticians contributed little to the family coffer. Instead, married women who worked in their homes prevented "girls who really need a salary from getting jobs." Hazel Bartholf thought that "married women with husbands that have fairly good salaries" owned home shops.[27] Similarly, shop owners in Topeka, Kansas's "business section" found that in their town of 65,000, they had twenty-eight legitimate beauty shops, "paying high rents," but as many as "70 housewives taking care of their homes and doing beauty work at odd times from 7 o'clock in the morning until 10 o'clock at night, if they wish, with no overhead for rent." Most likely, "their husbands are working at some good job downtown, perhaps for the railroad or some city job where we tax payers are paying him."[28] The neighborhood shop served no useful purpose, claimed Mrs. Esther Johnson, vice president of the Chicago Hairdressing Association. "In their own words," asserted Johnson, "they just do a little work for the girls in the neighborhood, and the girls leave whatever they feel its worth! Another word for that kind of work," she insisted was "pin money."[29]

Yet whether or not an operator was single or married, beauty operators who worked out of their homes or went door-to-door often provided considerable economic support for entire families. In New Brunswick, New Jersey, Josephine Nichols was "trying to conduct a small beauty business in [her] home, not for luxuries but to "help keep food in [her family's] mouths, as [her] husband is making only $10.00 a week as [a] night watchman." Nichols's business also kept her daughter in high school, and her family was proud to be "independent, and not ask for relief."[30] Similarly, a North Carolina woman operated a small beauty shop in her home and supported her younger sister and mother, who was "a widow, and unable to work."[31] Grace Brost, of Sunbury, Pennsylvania was just a girl of fourteen in 1933, but practically supported herself and her family by "putting in waves in the hair of my friends." In a letter to President Roosevelt, she told of her family's "bad luck." Her own father died before she was born, and her "step-father was a railroader but was recently hurt with result of an amputated leg and considerable injuries internally." "Thus he can not support us, [and] Mother cannot work as her health is very poor." Her brother was nineteen, but "he does not have good health due to [a] defect of his lung" even though he "tries to earn as much as he can." Nor did her step-brother seem to be a lot of help. Instead, she described him as someone "whom we must keep although he is 23 years and able to take care of himself." Doing finger waves, Brost found, allowed her to live somewhat comfortably. "I received enough money to clothe me," she explained, "and to keep me in school as well as to help my family a small amount."[32]

Of course, while many managed to turn meager resources into successful businesses during the toughest of times, their greatest challenge came not from the economic downturn per se but rather from hairdressing associations who were determined to use the NRA as a means of eliminating "illegitimate" businesses. In September 1933, one month after several organizations first met to propose a national hairdressing code in Washington, D.C., *Modern Beauty Shop*'s publisher, Charles J. Kutill, declared that "Now is the time for beauty shop owners to raise their prices on services," and put an end to "cut-price" competition and "sweatshop" conditions. In fact, he suggested that shop owners should not even wait "until your local organization decides on a price schedule." Instead, he urged "Do it yourself. You have a perfectly sound basis for raising prices" and, he argued, "the public expects it and will support you." *Modern Beauty Shop* suggested the following steps for success. First, "Sign the NRA code [and] Display the membership emblem in your shop." Second, "Put your operators on a 48 hour week [and] pay them a salary of at least $12 to $15 a week, according to the population stipulation in the President's code." Third, "Explain to your customers that your overhead has been increased by the necessary employment of extra help and increased wages, as well as increased cost of equipment and supplies." Fourth, "Tell your patrons to go forth and boast that they have their beauty work done at a shop that is not engaging in sweatshop practices but, on the contrary is supporting the President of the United States in bettering industrial conditions and stimulating re-employment."[33]

Raising the price of beauty services made little sense to most small shop owners, however. Miss Anne Buchanan insisted that in Norton, Virginia, "there is nothing here in the way of manufacturing, etc., and very little work going on, therefore, nothing to encourage the public to pay higher prices except for necessities." Nor did Buchanan feel as though she should be "forced to 'rob the public.'" While Buchanan distinguished herself from "girls who just 'picked up' hairdressing, [and] who will go from house to house and do finger waving for 15 c," she found herself at odds with most of the shop owners in her county who "wish to raise prices for the cheapest permanent to $5.00, and $1.00 for finger waving." "We have been threatened," Buchanan declared, and told "that they will put us out of business if we do not raise our prices." She had already raised the price of finger waves from thirty-five to fifty cents and charged four dollars for a permanent wave, but her "customers are mostly working girls who say they cannot possibly afford to pay more." Buchanan shortened hours and raised prices, but her business revenues were cut, "at least, in half."[34]

Similar conditions existed in the upper Midwest. Mrs. Agnes Plant wrote President Roosevelt to explain why a price increase would only harm small shop owners in Sauk Centre, Minnesota. "Here, in this farming community," she protested, "cream took a two ct drop last week," while "spring chickens are 5 and 6 cts a lb." At the same time that the NRA was demanding an increase in prices, "rural school teachers . . . [who] were getting $75–100 are staying this year for $35–$40, because, they know [what] kind of deal the farmers are getting." Many of the shops in Minneapolis and St. Paul, she found, regularly charged much higher prices, but that merely reflected urban life and the fact that many of "their regular customers . . . receive $18–20 a week." Because all consumer goods were cheaper in a small farming community "they should not call us 'cut-throats' when we put our prices in accordance to other things." Instead of gaining customer loyalty, Plant feared she would lose her business. Insisting on twenty-five cents for a vinegar or lemon rinse, she thought, "will only encourage our ladies to wash their hair at home" because "everyone knows half a lemon or 1 tablespoon of vinegar [is] 25 cts a gal." and she argued that five dollars "is likewise too much for a perm."[35]

The controversy over raising prices was not simply an issue of how much a lemon rinse or a gallon of vinegar cost, however; beauty operators complained that higher prices were unfair to working people and exceeded the boundaries of a "moral economy."[36] In other words, beauty operators, like the larger rural and working-class communities of which they were a part, had long understood that a fair and just price provided not only order and stability but maintained, in the words of beauty shop owners and consumers alike, a sense of decency amidst hard times. Mrs. Ines Conner noted that Kansas was "an agricultural state" and that conditions were so bad that "there were no crops here this year [1933], chickens are selling at 8 c, [and] butterfat at 16 c." As beauty operators, Conner declared, "we depend a great deal on the farmer trade." Of course, she objected to "cheap prices" but if a person "does not have the money," prices have to remain at a reasonable level. "Most of the shops in this state are small shops, [and employ] from 1–3 operators in a shop." "If these high prices go into effect," she warned, "these shops will have to lay off their help."[37] Mrs. R. A. Collins of Athens, Georgia, strongly concurred and argued that "as a rule" her customers were "working people" and unable to pay the "high prices" "high class" shops charged. "The material which goes into the Princess waive cost on average of 75 [cents] to $1.00" for which she charged $2.50 or what she called a "sufficient margin of profit." Raising prices, she felt would be "unfair to the public and allow a margin of profit nearing extortion." In her words, a dramatic increase in prices

> will result in choking out the smaller places which have heretofore catered to a class of trade which have not and will not go to places which are able to charge high prices and will be a detriment to business as well as inconvenience the public.[38]

As the experiences of these women suggest, the NHCA failed to understand the day-to-day struggles women in rural areas faced. In 1932, for example, *The American Hairdresser* assured its readership that "the Farm woman" would provide shop owners with a lucrative trade. According to an editor, the rural woman was "worth cultivating," because "she was able to turn her hand to pin money in many lines which the city woman would find practically impossible." "I have seldom met a farm woman or girl of beauty shop age who does not have a small producing garden, flock of chickens or some other means of making money" insisted the editor. And unlike the "town woman," who was "ridden by the rent, food, and light bills," the farm woman's "little income is hers."[39] To be sure, even girls with the most meager resources could on occasion scrape together enough money to frequent a small-town beauty shop. But farm families were unlikely to provide shops with a steady clientele. Instead, rural women often reserved a trip to the beauty shop for special occasions. Even in the 1990s, Angela Roberts found that in small Missouri towns "you've got some [customers] . . . from the country side," but they were "still in that old mind set" and visited the beauty shop only as a "special treat."[40]

During the Depression, a trip to the beauty shop was even more of a "special treat." Avis Bullock's "dad was barely hanging onto [their] 80-acre farm in Southern Missouri with the help of two mortgages" and all the "extra money" that her family could "scrape together." But Avis admitted that she was at a "self-conscious age" and thought she "needed a permanent in order to look nice before the new year in high school began." The only problem was that she did not have any money of her own. Instead her "oldest sister, Gwen, had a job cleaning people's homes" and offered to pay for the trip to the beauty shop. But living on a farm created other obstacles like trying to find a way to get from her family's farm to the nearby town. "My father," she recalled, "had never owned an automobile except for a Model T Ford, [but] in those days the owner of a car was, of necessity, his own mechanic." Usually "baling wire attached in the right place" and a "little patience" were all that a person needed, the latter of which Avis's father had very little. Once he sold the Model T, "he vowed that he would never own another car, therefore we had no transportation." "Early one morning, Gwen and I caught a ride the 10 miles into Golden City with a neighbor who hauled milk and cream to people in town." "The woman who gave me the permanent did a good job," Avis recalled, but she was "shocked" to discover her sister planned to walk the entire way home. While Avis proudly remembered "leaving the beauty salon with [her] beautiful new hairdo," she also never forgot that it was the first time she walked "10 miles in one stretch."[41]

Just as the NHCA had little understanding of everyday struggles of rural life, "industry leaders" also seemed to have little interest or knowledge regarding the problems endemic to the African-American beauty-culture industry. James Kefford, who was president of the Colored Beauty Shoppe Owners Association, which represented 1,500 beauticians in New York City and its surrounding suburbs, strongly opposed the idea of black and white hairdressers operating under the same code because of the differences in work. "Our work in the beauty-culture industry is so different to the work of white beauticians," Kefford argued, "that it would be disastrous for us to work under the same code." Part of that difference reflected the disparity between black and white wages. "The wages of the colored working girl at present are very small," insisted Kefford, "and if we have to increase beauticians' wages at this time the public will not be able to stand an increase in our prices and therefore it would throw a lot of colored operators who are now employed out of work." Only when the "servant girl" earns more than five or seven dollars a week, "could we make more money and pay more." Kefford asserted that the beauty culture industry was "providing more work for colored people than any other one industry in the United States," and "we are willing to do our part in the N.R.A. drive but we want conditions that we can prosper by and not suffer by."[42]

As Kefford's defense of the African-American hairdressing industry suggests, many beauty operators were often willing to compromise and do their part for the NRA. Mrs. Daisy Brown, for example, owned a "small residential shop" in Tampa, Florida, and had "been doing just about enough business to furnish a meager living" for herself and one employee. Brown admitted that her shop was "not beautiful" but was "kept clean and sanitary and only first class work is done here." In short, her shop was much more modest than "the high grade shops" that were "long established," "handsomely furnished," "have more modern equipment and more luxurious surroundings," and "have always charged higher prices." As a result, she was ambivalent about the establishment of a price code. On the one hand, she was proud to be a member of the NRA and wanted to "do [her] share toward recovery," but on the other hand, she worried that "we can not do it if [it meant being] thrown out to beg on the streets." She feared that an increase in prices would mean that she would be "put out of business" and "left with out any means of livelihood." Describing herself as an "older woman, too old to obtain employment anywhere," she had "nothing" else to turn to for support "even in the most meager way." Nor was she alone. "There are many other small shop owners in the same predicament" she explained, and "prices [should] be set according to the status of what they have to offer the public in the way of luxuries of furnishings." Rather than one price code, there should be three different classes with "the prices to fit the shop."[43]

Beauty operators in parts of the South were also willing to compromise. Annabell Criswell of Dallas, Texas, wrote on behalf of seventy-five "suburban" beauty shop owners who wanted to cooperate with the NRA, but "without sacrificing our little businesses, which are the sole means of support for us—many of whom are widows with families to care for." Criswell complained that the proposed price code for the Dallas area was "unfair and not truly representative." "We are patriotic [and] we want to cooperate in every way possible with Mr. Roosevelt," insisted Criswell, "but we need to be able to continue in business." "Instead of raising all former prices proportionately, [the code] only resulted in holding the current downtown shop prices and raising the suburban prices to meet their regular rates." For many shops this meant "an advance of 100% or more." This, she thought, was "unreasonable" and "business suicide for the small shops because our patrons cannot pay these advanced prices." According to Criswell, "a 50% advance in all prices" was "much more logical to us as it would not be prohibitive."[44]

In addition, some beauty operators simply could not understand why local hairdressing associations were unwilling to accept compromises. In Savannah, Georgia, for example, Elenora Christiansen complained that certain shop owners "would not give in one nickel from their very high prices." In a letter to Mrs. Roosevelt, Christiansen proudly described the "small beauty shop" in her home, which was not only kept "clean" but was quite "attractive" and freshly "painted pink and silver." "I cant understand why prices cant be made reasonable so the working girl can still have her finger wave etc. instead of being made so high that only the rich can enjoy it." "If some shops want to charge high prices, 'more power to them.'" "Better equipped shops," Christiansen thought, were certainly "entitled to higher prices than the small home shops." But she was concerned that if prices remained too high "only that class of shop can operate." "How can a girl earning ten to twelve dollars per week and the man with a family to support on a small salary fifteen to twenty-five dollars per week, give his wife and daughters money to have beauty work done if the prices are made so high." "You know today nearly every little shop girl has her hair fixed, and how unhappy she will be if she can't."[45]

Catering to wage-earning women involved more than keeping prices at a reasonable level, however. In order to meet the needs of the "shop girl" or factory worker, business hours also needed to remain flexible. For neighborhood shops, then, attempts to restrict hours were as problematic as any price code. Jane Brown, for example, lived in Kansas City, Missouri, and was upset that downtown shops were "trying to put a clause in the Code that will compel all shops to open at nine and close at six." Unlike the code's sponsors, Brown's customers were "working girls" who had to get their "beauty work done after business hours . . . between the hours of four and seven." If all shops must close early, she protested, "those girls will have to get their work done on their lunch hour in the down town shops. That is going to cause great hardship on all suburban shops owners."[46] Mrs. R. A. Collins also found that her "customers are as a rule, working people" who could not "make appointments during the hours from 9.00 A.M. to 5.00 P.M." and limited shop hours would ruin her business.[47] Similarly, a North Carolina woman explained that unlike the shops that insisted on closing at five in the afternoon, her shop did not "cater to the fashionable trade." Instead, her customers were mostly "girls who work at the sewing rooms, who can't come . . . until after the sewing rooms close [at] 6 o'clock in the afternoon" and only "a few [of her] customers . . . work in stores and come at meal hrs or after 5 o'clock in the afternoon." To make matters worse, she worried that if she failed to close at five o'clock, "I can't get a Blue Eagle & nobody will patronage me," and if "I can't take my class of trade when they are off from work . . . [I] will have to close up [any way] for lack of customers." Like many beauty operators, she asked the federal government to solve problems created by local associations. "I wish you would advise me how I can arrange to do my own work & get a Blue Eagle, for I think every body should do their part."[48]

Small shop owners were also unwilling to support codes which contained inherent class biases.[49] "I'm strong for the NRA," wrote Mrs. Leo Farmer of Dallas, Texas, "but we have a right to live, same as the higher ups." Farmer asked the NRA for "advice" for she feared she would lose her "Little [home] Beauty Shop" in the face of local opposition. She opened her shop only after her family's income "ha[d] been cut until [they] failed to meet the notes on [their] home and are about to lose it." But just as her business began to show signs of a profit, "the bigger shops have gotten up a code, forcing we little ones to sign it." It was obvious, she declared, that "they are trying to put we little ones out," by demanding that she double her prices. Adding insult to injury, the local association threatened her and insisted that if she did not cooperate she would be "subject to [a] $500 fine and 90 days in jail." In response, Farmer begged the NRA to respond quickly to her letter because she feared that the "head of this association" would call "again in the near future."[50]

Like Mrs. Leo Farmer, beauty operators across the country found their small neighborhood shops under attack all in the name of economic recovery. In Evansville, Indiana, for example, an operator who ran her shop with the help of her son heard "down town shops . . . making their brags [that] they are going to put the small shop out of business." "They are trying to get a Code through at so high that it will ruin all the shops except for the rich." Beauty operators in Evansville "made a good living through the depression with giving permanents at $1.50–$3.00." But the large downtown shops demanded that the minimum price for a permanent wave be five dollars, which this shop owner feared would "through me and my family on the city."[51] Mrs. Ines Conner thought that her "part of the country should be investigated before the Kansas Code is signed." "I am willing to do all in my power to cooperate with the N.R.A.," she insisted, "but if signing it means that I must raise my prices I cannot consciencely sign it." "Higher priced shops" in Wichita appointed all the members on code committees, she protested, and "you will find that it is not to hire more operators that these high prices are being

pushed, [for] there was no mention made of employing more operators but only of raising prices."[52]

In New York, the League of Master Beauticians was also leery of price codes and argued that "a small group of 'so-called' higher priced shops have been very active within the last several months," undermining the reputation of the small shop owner. According to the League, a certain "clique who consider themselves superior to the average beauty shop owner" had been circulating "false and misleading printed statements to the industry branding the popular priced beauty shop owners as 'cheap and unscrupulous.'" The League was particularly disturbed that "this group" had prepared a code "without [even] consulting with, or seeking the opinion or approval of, the majority shop owners of Greater New York." If the code passed, the League warned, it "will result in the elimination and wiping out of the popular priced beauty shops now serving the major portion of the general public."[53] The vice president of the Beauty Culture Code Association of Illinois maintained that the majority of Chicago's beauty shop owners "contest the right and authority of the National Hairdressers and Cosmetologist Association to present [a code]." "The vast majority of small, independent shops" often employ no extra help and "are the backbone of the industry," yet their interests were not represented. Instead a "monopoly" had been created that would "eliminate or oppress the small shops."[54]

As small neighborhood shops challenged the NHCA over price codes and hours of operation, gender distinctions further eroded the national association's legitimacy. In a letter to Mrs. Roosevelt, the American Cosmeticians Association insisted that the NHCA along with the proposed beauty shop code were not truly representative of the industry's needs. Instead, the NHCA "advocates the domination of this trade by their own group," a group the Association argued was "composed primarily of men who by chance have found their way in the Beauty shop trade as manufacturers, dealers and the owners of beauty shops, particularly in large communities." It seemed unreasonable to the American Association that men should attempt to control a "trade which consists of more than 90% women and is operated almost exclusively to serve women." The American Association and its membership throughout the United States, not to mention other female owners and operators the Association represented, "resent the entrance of men into this trade and regard them as intruders."[55]

Harold Demsey, an attorney who represented the American Association, found that beauticians "on all sides of Louisiana, . . . in Texas, in Arkansas, and in Mississippi . . . are outspoken in their prejudices against the National Association," which they referred to as "'an association for men' and an 'association of foreigners,'" for which these female operators had no patience. Indeed, Demsey had no idea "how or where a code committee of the National Association could obtain local support." In his home state of Louisiana, Demsey knew of only one member. "A chapter of the National was attempted here several times," he recalled, "but they couldn't get the half-dozen or so necessary to form the chapter." As a result, "News of the recognition of the National Association as the temporary authority of the trade had not been well received" and created as much controversy as one would expect to find "if the Barber Shop Code were to be placed in the hands of a bunch of women."[56]

Because the NHCA seemed to have little concern for the neighborhood shop, many operators often ignored local associations, initially signing code agreements and adjusting wages and hours accordingly, but soon reverting back to previous business practices. Mrs. Catherine J. Danner, chairman of the Hairdressers Association of Elk, Cameron, and Potter Counties, Pennsylvania, complained that several beauty operators in Emporium "have in their display window[s] big blue eagles from last year, and they are all working any and all hours." It was unfair that "they are allowed to have the eagle displayed [while] breaking the hours we voted on." Indeed, Danner discovered that many operators were "putting in 70 to 100 hrs a week and cutting prices or otherwise going right opposite to the recovery program." In addition, they seemed to have little success imposing restricted hours because operators "will take enough appointments before closing time to keep them busy for hours." At least the barber, noted Danner, had the decency to lock the doors and pull his blind down while he finished ten or fifteen customers. "But Mrs. Bateman, [another beauty operator] don't even pull down the blind—she works so anyone can see her working."[57]

Blue Eagles, Neighborhood Shops

Of course the small shop owner was not the only one guilty of ignoring local codes. In fact, those who were most effective in manipulating the NRA controlled the greatest resources. In Alabama, for example, beauty operators found themselves competing with Mr. Hugh Conner, who owned "large cotton mills all over the State." "Up until the time of raising the labor's wages at the cotton mills those girls worked for $7.20 a week," complained Leta May Johnson, "then when he was compelled under the N.R.A. to raise wages He immediately opens Beauty shops to get the returns from that too." According to Johnson, "there are four girls trying to make their living in this town in small shop's, [but] Conner cuts them off by compelling his employes to patrinize his beauty shops and cutting the prices and making and keeping this beauty shop open until 8 o'clock pm. when we are asked to close at 6 pm." Beauty shop owners were especially upset to find some of the cotton mill employees, who already worked eight hours, earning extra income in Conner's beauty shop. "It is not fair," declared Johnson. "Large cotton plant owners could do well to confine their supply to the cotton mills instead of crushing smaller places of business."[58]

Beauty schools were also creating problems for large and small shops alike. Beauty schools not only profited from cheap student labor but used the apprenticeship system to justify cheap prices. The apprenticeship system long posed a problem for many beauticians as soon as it became popular. The Depression only made matters worse. William E. Trull owned a ten-booth beauty salon in Wichita, Kansas, and noted that in theory the "primary purpose" of a beauty school was to "teach students the art of cosmetology," but in reality he found beauty schools were "nothing short of slavery." "Usually the course of study covers a total of 1000 hours of work," and according to Trull, "the majority of this work is practical in that the students work on subjects willing to have a beginner work on them." It did not take long, however, for "students [to] become very good at their work [and] in a few weeks then the school begins to charge for the work." Of course, the entire proceeds went to the school. Consequently, beauty schools required many students to work from six to ten hours per day, which Trull insisted, causes "hardship on the regular shop but enslaves the girls doing the work." Trull was convinced that in order to increase profits, schools would often single out their best students and "hold them over from one to three months." Trull even knew of one student who "was working from six to ten hours per day bringing into the school fund from five to ten dollars per day. She had completed her required work or number of hours." But the school would not let her graduate because the "girl's work was very unsatisfactory;" therefore "she would be required to take two or three months of work," which meant that she would continue to make money for the school without receiving any wages in return.[59]

Despite complaints about the NRA and its inherent weaknesses, the NHCA still described its initial success as the "DAWN OF A BRIGHTER DAY." Indeed, the NRA breathed new life into the NHCA and galvanized affiliated organizations that had disbanded in the early days of the Depression. Above all, the NHCA insisted that the NRA had secured its "position as the 'Voice of Cosmetology in the Nation,'" a voice that would not only govern the organization of beauty shops and schools, but also help define the image of the industry. Since the early 1920s, the NHCA along with various other reform organizations had pushed for stronger rules to regulate the industry in an attempt to protect the consumer and improve working conditions. But controlling prices, wages, business hours, and consumer safety was not simply about improving the condition of the industry; it was also part of a broader attempt to clean up the industry's image. This meant eliminating the kitchen beautician and all the "problems" associated with her shop in order to cultivate a different and a more professional image.[60]

The professional image the NHCA embraced did indeed exclude women. *The American Hairdresser* characterized the ideal hairdresser as a well-educated businessman with an eye for artistry, yet well grounded in scientific training:

> He is, first, a genus of artists. . . . He creates coiffures [which require] a sense of art values in both balances and lines [as well as] coloring of hair and skin. . . . He must have scientific accomplishments. . . . He reconditions hair, scalp and skin and must be familiar with their structure; his information must include anatomy and chemical composition. . . . He

[also] uses machinery, and the elements of steam and electricity in many forms, and last, but not least he is a businessman. . . . His activities include over-the-counter sales in the manner of any merchandiser.

According to NHCA, "any single one of these activities" should have legitimized the trade and "definitely [kept] the field out of the menial class."[61] But in order to reclaim a position for hairdressers in the world of white-collar work, it was clear that the NHCA intended to meet definitions of professionalism, which were exclusively male and middle-class, definitions that had long excluded women from other occupations.[62]

The kind of professionalism the NHCA strived to emulate, then, stood in bold contrast to the neighborhood shop which was not only a female institution, but steeped in the daily rituals of working-class life. How could the NHCA, for example, achieve any semblance of professionalism when investigators, upon entering a typical neighborhood shop in the Bronx, "tripped over" the beauty operator's "toddling baby and a puppy," who were playing together "in the dark entrance," while finding the kitchen sink used to rinse hair "filled with dirty dishes." Like many neighborhood businesses, this shop "occupied three front rooms of [the owner's] apartment in a tenement above a bakery" and thus violated middle-class notions of family privacy. It was tiny, "every bit of available space was filled with waiting patrons," and "there was no chair for the [investigator], but no one cared." Here the working-class customers were mainly immigrants, and the sights and sounds of the Italian community filled the shop. A "radio blared 'hot numbers'" in the background while "Everyone was engaged in a cross conversation that included operators." Despite the NHCA's insistence that gossip was bad for business, "admittedly," the investigator found that "the atmosphere was very friendly and club-like," and "the patrons, [who] were largely Italian . . . seemed quite satisfied," just like a "big, happy family." Even though the investigator defined the Bronx shop owner as a "skillful hostess," she insisted that "no one with her ideas of sanitation should be called a [hairdresser]."[63]

Above all, the neighborhood shop with its working-class and ethnic character was inextricably bound to dirt and disease.

According to the investigator, the Italian woman often ignored NHCA sanitation guidelines and refused to wash her hands: "When a customer wants me to wash my hands, [then] I wash them. I even wash the instruments." But even after "she dipped her hands in the finger bowl and wiped them with a dubious little napkin," the investigator noticed that the owner was just going through the motions. Her hands remained "blackish" while "her arms and uniform were splattered with black dye, even her nose showed a tracery of black dots." Perhaps most disturbing from the investigator's standpoint was the owner's insistence on "retraining" beauty school graduates who, in the shop owner's own words, were "nuts on this here sanitation." One of the shop's newest employees who graduated "from a big school . . . wanted to wash her hands and sterilize the combs, brushes, towels, and everything all the time." The routine was apparently causing problems in the shop as another operator "got awful sore," recalled the owner. But after a while, the shop owner was pleased to say that her recent hire "got over that school nonsense . . . and now she's the best worker in the place."[64]

The kitchen beautician with her dollar perms, twenty-five cent finger waves, and unconventional methods directly challenged notions of professionalism and middle-class respectability. But the investigator's disdain for this neighborhood beauty parlor was not simply a matter of cheap perms; she was more disturbed with the nature of the shop and the owner's attitude. For the Italian beauty operator living in the Bronx, respectability did not come from the NHCA, but from the community. For example, gossip, rather than being seen as somehow unprofessional, was expected and considered an important part of the beauty shop and community life. Even *The American Hairdresser*, while it criticized social networks that defined beauty shop culture, admitted that gossip created strong emotional bonds between operators and their customers, suggesting that the beauty shop, no matter how small or how cluttered, was a crucial working-class institution.[65] Moreover, many female association leaders voiced a conscious rejection of the NHCA's definition of professionalism. The American Cosmetician's Association, a female-dominated organization, admitted that "in Europe the leaders of this Trade are men and are called Hairdressers; but in America, the leaders of this

Trade are women and they resent being called Hairdressers and have adopted the terms: cosmetician, beautician, beauty culturist, etc., in fact, any term to get away from the European methods and to be distinctly American."[66] Mrs. Nellis Ramsey, president of the Kansas State Association, liked the "good old American word 'operator,'" rather than fancier terms like "cosmetologist," "cosmetician," or even "beautician," suggesting that it was the elitism she linked to Eurocentric hairdressing associations that angered midwestern beauty operators.[67]

But in challenging professionalism, the neighborhood shop also blurred the lines designed to maintain rigid racial distinctions. Barbara Melosh argues that because of women's "second-sex" status, the notion of a woman's profession was and remains a contradiction in terms. Nursing, for example, "cannot be a profession because most nurses are women."[68] Like nursing, hairdressing had a difficult time maintaining a professional image because of the disproportionate numbers of women in the occupation and because of the atmosphere investigators found in many beauty shops. But in the hairdressing industry, professionalism was not simply an issue of gender. "Coolie wages," "sweat-shop" conditions and "slave labor," according to the NHCA, resulted from the unregulated growth of the unsanitary neighborhood shops, which had cheapened the industry and undermined professionalism. As a result, hairdressing was not classified with doctors and dentists, white-male occupations, but with domestics and porters, jobs disproportionately filled by African Americans. In other words, professionalism was based as much on race as on gender and class and just as industry leaders excluded working-class women from definitions of professionalism, so too were African Americans and other non-white workers. According to Manning Marable, "the Black Sharecropper in the South became a blue collar or service worker in the East Coast and Middle West," and even though "the bulk of black business activity moved with the massive migration North. . . . The Golden Years of Black business [1919–1929]" were also "the period of the most extensive racial segregation." In other words, while African Americans moved into many professions, white Americans continued to view the black professional as a contradiction in terms.[69] Non-white labor, then, remained inextricably bound to service

116   work, cast in terms of servility, linked to disease and dirt, and most assuredly distinct from even the least prestigious of white occupations.

In his study of Milwaukee, Joe William Trotter also found that African Americans "almost exclusively, entered the city's expanding domestic, personal service, and common laborer positions." The Plankinton House, for example, "was the largest and oldest of these employers of black labor. Afro-Americans worked there and in similar establishments as bellboys, cloakroom and washroom attendants, cooks, maids, porters, waiters, and so on." Moreover, Trotter argues that only waiters were able to "transcend somewhat 'the stigma of servility' attached to this type of work and gain modest opportunities for advancement." Domestic and personal service employment also consistently paid the lowest wages. And as opportunities in industrial cities expanded, it seemed that "wherever the work was hot, dirty, low-paying, and heavy, black men could be found."[70]

By the early years of the Depression, black men "lost the bulk of their industrial foothold, [and] Afro-American women found it necessary to seek domestic and personal service work in greater numbers," occupations which fit popular racial stereotypes. In contrast, the number of white women employed in domestic service dramatically decreased in number. Between 1900 and 1930, the number of white women working in domestic service decreased by half, while the percentage of white women working in industry also dropped from 33 to 21 percent. At the same time, "where the black females worked in close proximity to whites, the work was stratified along racial lines." In Milwaukee's Schroeder Hotel, for example, African-American women "operated the freight elevator, scrubbed the floors, and generally performed the most disagreeable maid's duties." In contrast, "white women worked the passenger elevator, filled all clerical positions, and carried out light maid's duties."[71]

Similarly, in white-owned beauty shops, racial distinctions were often reinforced through occupational definitions and wages. The Texas Association of Accredited Beauty Culturists, for example, was particularly concerned that the federal government classified beauticians with domestic labor and expected beauty shops to pay maids 75 percent of an operator's wage. The Texas as-

Blue Eagles, Neighborhood Shops

sociation explained that "this is way too much" because "in the South and Southwest," they hired "only Negro and Mexican help." "Our white girls, to a great extent, would starve before they would serve as maids," insisted the association. In fact, white beauty shop owners thought that the maids they hired to clean their shops should only receive half their "present salary" because "the Negro and the Mexican laborers cannot stand prosperity; they are not appreciative, and few of them try to better their condition." An increase in pay "would only spoil them and would thereby work a hardship in the homes as well as in business." "The Beauty Operator," the association claimed, "is an artist in her own right, and we believe her wages are low enough but we certainly do not believe the maid is entitled to 75% as much money for her services and plead for her some relief from this over estimate of her value."[72]

Escaping domestic service work also meant disassociating oneself from the stigma attached to such jobs. Euro-American hairdressing associations understood that professionalism ensured racial distinctions and the government's careless system of classification disturbed them as much as the low wages and long hours. In Jacksonville, Florida, for example, Virginia Williams, owner of Betsy Ross Beauty Shop, wrote President Roosevelt asking him to give "proper recognition and rating for [her] profession." While attending Florida's state convention, Williams was "astonished" that Washington offices categorized her work with the "servant class," which included "charwomen" and "laundresses." "This is deplorable considering the high type of people now employed in our shops," Williams insisted.[73] And in Dover, New Jersey, Mary Tirella, owner of The Mayflower Beauty Shop and member of the New Jersey Hairdressing Association, found "a great difference between a domestic and a Beautician" and complained that in New Jersey "we beauticians are classed, not as professionals, but as domestics."[74] Similarly, on the West Coast a hairdresser who worked at Jim's Beauty Studio on Hollywood's Sunset Boulevard was distraught to learn that the NRA had classed beauticians with "Delivery Men, Drivers, Dishwashers." Instead, he insisted that a "Beauty Parlor Operator really performs individual and personal service, and should be classed the same as a Dentist, Doctor or Chiropractor." The shop's manager also argued that a "beauty parlor was not the same as a Barber Shop where the Barber yells 'NEXT.'" Instead, Jim's Studio made individual appointments and specialized their services to fit the needs of famous clients such as Salley Eilers and Mae West. "The classification . . . as it stands at present," he protested, was "hurting an operator and also the business."[75]

In the Midwest, complaints over the classification of the hair-dressing industry were also bound to issues of race. St. Clair Drake and Horace R. Cayton's study of Chicago reveals that African Americans in 1930 were "doing a disproportionately large amount of the city's servant work, and a disproportionately small amount of 'clean work.'" "Clean work on the eve of the Depression," argues Drake and Cayton, included "professional, proprietary, managerial, and clerical work, [and] was almost a white monopoly." Only 2 percent of Chicago's black population could be included in "Chicago's large white-collar class," and "those few Negroes who did 'clean work,'" they argued, "were almost entirely confined to the Black Ghetto and were dependent upon wage-earning masses for a livelihood, or upon the ability of white people to pay for their services as entertainers."[76] While the Chicago and Illinois Hairdressing Associations maintained that there were key educational differences between hairdressing and service work, they seemed well aware of racially defined occupational distinctions. Both associations were appalled that the NRA's legal department, under the auspices of the Blanket Code, had placed "BEAUTY OPERATORS IN THE SAME CATEGORY AS DISHWASHERS JANITORS PORTERS [and] WATCHMEN."[77] Drake and Cayton's study revealed that many service occupations such as janitorial work had long been considered "Negro Jobs" and although that was changing in the face of immigration, African-American men retained a "monopoly" in certain occupations such as that of porter. "'George,' the Negro Pullman porter," Drake and Cayton argue, "is an American institution."[78] It was this consciousness of race that led hairdressing associations to "RESPECTFULLY ASK THAT BEAUTY OPERATORS BE PLACED IN A CLASS BEFITTING THEIR PROFESSIONAL EDUCATION AND TRAINING."[79]

Thus the classification the federal government was attempting to establish undermined the "psychological wage" upon which many white hairdressers based their identity.[80] "It must

be remembered," insisted W. E. B. Du Bois, "that the white
groups of laborers, while they received a low wage, were com-
pensated in part by a sort of public deference and titles of courtesy because they were white."[81] A hairdressing code that
treated beauty culture as a profession, then, would not simply
raise wages; it would help define the trade and preserve a sense
of respectability based on whiteness regardless of class. To be
sure, various white hairdressing associations and individuals
argued in support of regulation because it would improve conditions for the sake of both worker and consumer. But they
were nevertheless consumed with an unfailing desire to uplift
their industry and reassert racial distinctions that separated
hairdressing from other service occupations associated with
African-American and immigrant labor.

Because the hairdressing industry was rigidly divided by race,
the NHCA could completely ignore the dynamics of the black
hairdressing industry. When African-American women appeared
in white-owned beauty shops, they worked almost exclusively as
maids, reassuring white beauty operators that their work, no matter how demanding, was more respectable. Moreover, white
working-class beauty operators' rejection of NHCA standards of
professionalism did not suggest a lack of racial consciousness. Instead, Jim Crow and segregation ensured white neighborhood
shop owners that they would enjoy an identity and business
based on the politics of racial exclusion. Even as African Americans challenged these racial barriers, the Depression nevertheless
served as a reminder to white hairdressing associations that they
failed to meet their own definitions of professionalism. The Blue
Eagle, then, not only stood as a symbol of patriotism, it also held
out the hope that the professionalization of whiteness would
bring respectability to a trade whose classification and color were
not clearly defined.

Governmental efforts to regulate the beauty-culture industry
came to a swift end once the NRA was declared unconstitutional,
but the struggle to establish a code revealed a rigid division in the
industry. Although the kitchen beautician and the neighborhood
shop with one or two operators were recognized as the backbone

of the industry, they were also a thorn in the side of the NHCA. Indeed, the Chicago man who visited Laura Wernsman and her sister and insisted that neither cut their neighbor's hair was most likely not a fake, but rather someone who saw the two girls and their business as a dangerous threat to an industry still struggling to define itself. The establishment of the NRA codes was the opportunity for which large shop owners and industry associations had been looking to expand their efforts to professionalize the occupation—a process that had begun in the 1920s. NRA regulations that raised wages and established what the NHCA considered appropriate hours of operation not only challenged the door-to-door hair presser and the neighborhood shops that operated at all hours of the day but also targeted the types of shops that industry associations believed were guilty of mixing unsafe hair products, ignoring basic sanitation guidelines, and using worn out and unsafe equipment. In short, supporting the NRA meant the elimination of the working-class shops the NHCA labeled as dangerous and claimed were undermining the legitimacy of the industry and the professional image it embraced. As such the kitchen beautician was not only corrupting the industry because of her make-shift beauty shop, its informal atmosphere, and her willingness to gossip. Her working-class shop was also responsible for the close association of the beauty shop with domestic work and other service industries that African Americans and other non-white workers disproportionately occupied.

The demise of the NRA did not, of course, convince the NHCA to accept the small neighborhood shop. But World War II and the expansion of the industry in the postwar period did create a more flexible understanding of business and professionalism. As the economic strain of the Depression exacerbated the tension surrounding wage rates and hours of operation, the affluence of the post-World War II period helped reduce it. Indeed, the beauty industry's dramatic growth transformed the make-shift beauty shop into a more acceptable institution that further encouraged its development as a community institution and redefined to a limited degree the meaning of professionalism.

4

"Growing Faster Than the Dark Roots on a Platinum Blonde"

The Golden Years of the Neighborhood Shop

By the 1940s and '50s, Lulline Long of Birmingham, Alabama, was a financial success. During the Depression, Long, "with a suitcase on her hip," went door-to-door selling hair preparations, cosmetics, and toiletries to African-American women, saving the Cannolene Cosmetic Company and Distribution Store from financial disaster. Rebuilding the business from the bottom up, Long opened her first beauty shop in her house, and, according to her husband Robert, it was there where she also taught beauty culture and "did hair—what you call the marcel (wave)." Her business quickly outgrew its humble beginnings, and soon she owned and operated a two-story building which housed the Cannolene store, a salon, and a beauty school. Her husband remembered that while Parker High School girls from "up the street . . . would stop by to get their hair done," Lulline would also "bring boys in off the street and cut their hair for free—just so she could get a chance to talk to them." Robert recalled that this gave her the opportunity to "tell them about staying out of trouble, about making something of themselves, and about God." Long's business success not only allowed her the time to offer free haircuts and advice, but the financial wherewithal needed to maintain an unexpected library in the back of her beauty shop which offered an "extensive collection" of African-American history books as well as "other treasures."[1]

In many ways, Lulline Long's success in beauty culture was quite common in the decades following the Depression. Like Long, beauticians across the country used their shops for the good of their communities, organizing in support of America's war effort and in opposition to Jim Crow. But the beauty shop during the postwar period and the 1950s and '60s in particular, is perhaps best known for its dramatic economic expansion, a time when visits to the neighborhood beauty shop became an important ritual. Like Long, whose business began by going door-to-door and then developed into a two-story building that housed her salon, beauty school, and store, the beauty culture industry experienced unprecedented growth. Part of this expansion was simply a reflection of a vibrant U.S. economy, which provided women with more money to spend on beauty needs, services, and products. But it was also about style and the role beauty shops would come to play in the everyday lives of American women. Even during the Depression and war, beauty processes and products continued to sell, but with the end of World War II, practicality seemed less of a concern as simple "victory coiffures" began competing with more elaborate hairstyles that required constant attention and frequent visits to the beauty shop.[2]

The growing demand for beauty services during the postwar years affected the industry in unexpected ways. First, it led to a shortage of women willing to work as beauty operators and thus a crisis for the hairdressing industry as a never-ending array of hair products brought this labor shortage into sharp relief. Second, it helped legitimize the small neighborhood shop. Eager to sell their products to customers and operators alike, manufactures and trade journals helped legitimize the small, seemingly unprofessional shop by defining it in terms of domestic needs. Thus unlike preceding decades, when industry leaders derided the in-home shop as the bane of the industry, by the 1940s and 1950s, small-time operators had become the model for an industry looking to meet unprecedented consumer demands. Indeed, a booming economy and labor-intensive hair styles meant enough space for both the fashionable downtown salon and the modest neighborhood shop. Moreover, the skill and time required to care for the complicated bouffants and beehives that became popular in the postwar era meant that fewer clients were necessary to establish and maintain a successful business. The neighborhood shop, which had long offered the kind of flexibility wage-earning women, housewives, and mothers had insisted was necessary, now fit neatly into the profit equation industry leaders envisioned—all of which made the postwar decades a golden age for the small neighborhood beauty parlor.

During the Depression, the NHCA had complained incessantly about the abundance of female operators, claiming they were undermining prices and wages and the industry's professional image. With World War II, an entirely new set of problems emerged. Instead of there being too many operators, suddenly there were too few. Many beauty operators simply left the trade for higher paying jobs made available during the war. In 1943, for example, the auto industry, which had boasted an almost exclusively male work force before the war, now had women in one-fourth of its positions. Similarly, on the eve of America's involvement in World War II, the percentage of female electrical workers was slightly over 30 percent. By 1944, almost half the work force was female. While a sexual division of labor ensured that women's wages would remain significantly lower than their male counterparts (approximately at 66 percent of men's wage rates), those war industries that were particularly dependent on female substitution offered women wages that came much closer to men's hourly rates. In radio manufacturing, which employed significant numbers of women, the hourly rate for women was seventy-six cents, while men received ninety-nine cents. In auto manufacturing, the wage differential was even smaller. In 1944, women working in Michigan's auto plants received 90 percent of the rates paid to men.[3]

In response to the labor shortage, the NHCA actually found itself, for the first time, attempting to relax rather than restrict licensing laws to increase the pool of beauty workers. In 1942, Hazel Koslay, editor of *The American Hairdresser*, informed her readers that "Numerous schools have had to close their doors 'for the duration' and beauty salons are wondering whether this will bring about a serious shortage of operators and a painfully high wage scale."[4] One year later, *The American Hairdresser* declared that a "manpower shortage is now one of the most critical topics on the home front of the war program" and suggested granting "temporary licenses," especially for women moving from a state that lacked licensing requirements to a state that had specific laws.[5] Although there were still fears that reducing standards would allow "incompetents to enter the field," something had to be done to keep the nation's 83,000 beauty salons in operation.[6] Thus various states granted temporary licenses to beauty workers who moved from one state to another and asked women to come out of retirement by offering to automatically reinstate their licenses. And for those just being trained in the field, *The American Hairdresser* suggested seeking work immediately in any area they had mastered. "While most people agree that all-round training is the best," Hazel Koslay, reminded her readers that "this is a time when compromises must be accepted."[7]

During the war, the hairdressing industry also seemed particularly concerned that the beauty shop find its patriotic niche. Throughout the early 1940s there were rumors that the government would close beauty shops, and some beauty editors even questioned the necessity of beauty parlors during a time of such crisis.[8] Hazel Kozlay admitted that the beauty business could not be classified as an "essential" industry. Yet in her words, hairdressing deserved "a prominent place in the supplementary lists, which included industries necessary to maintain the war industries and to maintain civilian life."[9] In a letter published in *The American Hairdresser*, Mildred Coldwell, of Yorkshire, England, made it clear why the beauty shops deserved a "prominent place." According to Coldwell, "Your customers will expect you to be the essence of cheerfulness under even the most trying conditions, and also a fountain of knowledge with regard to war news."[10]

Like their English counterparts, American shop owners were expected to do their part to help their customers, communities, and businesses cope with the crisis, and many did. In Hastings, Missouri, for example, hairdressers put on a scrap drive that led to the collection of three truckloads of useful materials. In turn, the money they collected from the sale of scrap material was "turned over to the Community War Chest."[11] Maude Gadsen of New York City organized the Beauticians Volunteer Corps in 1941 to "help in the war effort." The Corps sold "$4 million worth of war bonds and stamps [and] . . . held a parade down Seventh Avenue with 500 beauticians marching in honor of Dory Miller, the first Black man from New York to fall in the war."[12] In St. Louis, beauty parlors also helped "speed up" the sale of war stamps, but in this case the shop owner used anti-Japanese sentiment. Gladys Kidd, owner of Co-Ed Beauty Salon, invented "a clever [g]ame" designed to sell war stamps, something she nicknamed the "Twelve Little Japs." It seems that when Kidd found out that it only took twenty-five cents to buy twelve bullets, she not only bought a stamp book containing four twenty-five cent stamps each for every operator she employed but informed them that "every additional stamp you put in the book will kill twelve Japs." Now rather than spending money "foolishly," she boasted, her operators buy a stamp and proudly announce in the shop, "I killed 12 Japs today." The "game" was quite successful, and one of the operators even reported having been able to "buy three bonds since the game started."[13]

Hairdressers like the larger beauty culture industry of which they were a part also focused on the woman war worker's femininity and argued that beauty was an important means of maintaining morale on the home front. As Kathy Peiss notes, "the attractive made-up woman of the 1940s bespoke the 'American Way of Life' and a free society worth defending."[14] Similarly, the NHCA insisted that the nation's morale rested on the shoulders of women and "good grooming was an essential factor."[15] At the same time, war manufacturers and Uncle Sam were particularly concerned that Rosie-the-Riveter retain her femininity, especially as she moved into "men's jobs." In some occupations, manufacturers redefined traditionally male jobs to ensure gender distinctions. Recruiting pamphlets often pointed out the "similarity between squeezing orange juice and the operation of a small drill press," or they compared peeling potatoes to burring and filing.[16] Manufacturers even began to emphasize the importance of good grooming to further reassure skeptics who feared that changes in women's work would undermine American womanhood and morale. Thus as women took over traditionally male occupations during the war, beauty shops found their patriotic place. As one Clairol shampoo advertisement put it: "Beauty Shops have a war job, too" and that job was maintaining feminine beauty even during the toughest of times.[17] To encourage women workers to spend precious time and money in beauty shops, *The American Hairdresser* suggested that business owners use a red, white, and blue color scheme in window displays and patriotic themes like "Be Brave Be Beautiful" to capture the attention of the casual passerby and make crucial connections between beauty, patriotism, and victory. Beauty shop window displays would not only inform the "war worker that you are conscious of her needs and are equipped to satisfy them," but also the housewife and student who may not have realized that "keep[ing] up their appearance" was vital to "civilian morale."[18] The NHCA even mailed beauty shops patriotic sales kits complete with "poster, window streamers, pledge cards, register stickers, coin cards and special tags for each employee to wear, all bearing the slogan 'Be the Woman Behind the Man, Behind the Gun.'"[19]

Of course, trips to the beauty shop were not cast simply as an issue of femininity, but also as a matter of practicality. Defense work, *The American Hairdresser* insisted, demanded a tidy, short-cropped hairstyle. "Long, untidy 'glamour' styles are out, and short, easy-to-manage bobs are in fact becoming an absolute necessity."[20] Whether women were working in hospitals or factories, "Victory Coiffures," the journal explained, needed to be "short and serviceable" yet always "neat and feminine." While short hair was easier to care for, the styles featured in *The American Hairdresser* were also versatile and "attractively feminine because the men in the service are definite in their demands that the girls back home remain feminine."[21]

In order to give women the styles they needed, beauty operators followed customers into their new surroundings. At Missouri's Fort Leonard Wood, Uncle Sam built a beauty shop at the "army training center for a detachment of WACs stationed there."[22] At the same time, the WAC post at Fort Des Moines, which opened in 1942, found that within a year it had to double its number of beauty shop employees to meet the demands of 200 customers who made appointments each day. Permanents were particularly "high on the list of favored services" because, according to the shop owner, permanents provided the "firm foundation" a hair style needed "if it is to be expected to last throughout the rigorous activity of WAC training." A lot of women also visited the shop for cutting and styling "because of the Army regulation that hair must be well above the collar and also because the WACs have learned that short hair is the easiest to take care of."[23]

Beauty shops also followed women into the factory. Not only did manufacturers claim that beauty shops helped attract female workers, but also did wonders for morale—meaning of course worker efficiency. Thanks to the opening of a factory beauty shop, "everybody's satisfied at the Republic Drill and Tool Company's large war plant in Chicago." In 1943, 80 percent of the employees were women, and according to the trade journal, "the war workers on the 'swing' and 'graveyard' shifts who found their unusual working hours incompatible with the working hours of the city's beauty shops can now have their shampoos and sets before they go to work in the evening, or before they leave for home in the morning." Company executives were pleased with the factory beauty shop "because they are convinced that beauty aids boost morale and that good grooming promotes health and safety for their employees." The beauty shop's owner, Maria Tolva, was also "happy because her appointment book is full and her cash register is ringing." Tolva had twelve operators working in the shop, who offered "the girls new ideas in hair cuts, and styles, designed to keep their tresses out of the machinery." They also gave factory hands make-up tips. "Protective make up and hand care," she insisted, was of the utmost importance "for beauty-conscious lady machinists."[24]

Ironically, at a time when women wage earners were desperate for child care facilities, factories often seemed more willing to sponsor beauty shops.[25] A beauty shop, for example, opened in a Ferndale, Michigan, war plant where profit-minded manufacturers insisted it would help reduce absenteeism. The Michigan plant manufactured "over 120 precision air craft engine parts" and on March 15, 1943, celebrated the opening of its own beauty shop. The beauty salon was large, with surroundings and furnishings as "fine as those found in many exclusive salons." In fact, the company president, N. A. Woodworth, considered in-house beauty services a "great factor in reducing absenteeism." "Extensive research," Woodworth insisted, "has revealed that many of our young ladies in working seven days a week find it impossible to secure those personal items and treatments which have become a necessity to every American woman." The beauty shop even operated around the clock to meet the needs of 3,000 employees, and appointments were made for women workers both before and after their shifts. To encourage "good attendance," the company also offered cash credits, which after twelve weeks of continued work could be exchanged for beauty services or cosmetics. In addition, the company was planning to give extra time off for hair appointments to employees with outstanding records. The entire plan, insisted the company owner, was designed to raise employee morale and ensure high productivity.[26]

The continued popularity of the beauty shop during the war was no doubt a product of patriotism and the potential concerns that accompanied working in a war plant. But they also thrived because of the scarcity of other consumer goods. Defense production meant there was little in the way of durable items available for purchase. Even though some items like hair pins became scarce because of metal shortages, forcing hairdressers to make do with homemade supplies and recycled products, beauty shops did not suffer the same kind of economic woes that brought other industries to a halt. Indeed, with fewer consumer goods available and unprecedented numbers of women in good paying industrial jobs, women found they had extra money and nothing on which to spend it. Beauty shops thus seemed to attract consumer dollars that could have gone towards the purchase of refrigerators, washing machines, and other goods and supplies put on hold for the duration of the war.[27]

Of course not all beauticians found themselves working just in support of the war effort. With World War II, African Americans once again faced the contradiction of fighting facism abroad as they faced unrelenting racism at home. Thus it is not surprising that as troops were sent to Europe, Asia, and North Africa, many black Americans embraced the Double V Campaign and A. Philip Randolph's threatened march on Washington to protest racial discrimination in employment and the military, a protest movement

hope and pessimism, support and detachment."[28] One of the most
dedicated and outspoken black leaders and beauticians challenging discrimination during the war was Marjorie Stewart Joyner.
Throughout her life and throughout most of twentieth century,
she committed herself to the advancement of African Americans
and beauty-culture. In the 1920s, she helped write the first Illinois beauty-culture laws, and while working as the Chairwoman
of the Chicago *Defender* Charities, she helped raise food and clothing for the needy. In the 1930s, she continued her charity work,
wrote an instructional manual for beauty-culture students, and
sued the Burlington Rock Island Railroad for their Jim Crow policies.[29] During World War II, Joyner continued to challenge the
status quo by running a Service Men's Center in Chicago. The center provided both social events and supplies for African-American soldiers at a time when black soldiers, like their World War I
predecessors, were being attacked by violent mobs. In fact, during 1943 alone, there were 242 "racial battles" in 47 cities, many
of which involved black soldiers.[30]

One of Joyner's greatest contributions was her commitment to
improving educational opportunities for African Americans, especially for beauty culturists. In the 1930s and '40s, this commitment to education was realized when she combined efforts with
Mary Mcleod Bethune, who, with the help of Eleanor Roosevelt,
established the Bethune-Cookman College in Daytona Beach,
Florida. According to Joyner, the women toured the country together to promote education and Walker products. "I was working for Madam Walker, [and] Dr. Bethune was trying to get black
people a higher education." In 1945, Joyner founded the United
Beauty School Owner Teaching Association (UBSOTA) and the
Alpha Chi Pi Omega Sorority and Fraternity in Washington, D.C.
Joyner's commitment to higher education and to her profession
inspired her to make UBSOTA the first beauty-culture organization to require college credits for membership.[31]

With the war's end, America's contradictions only became
more visible. Here was a nation, as Manning Marable points out,
that found the crimes of the Third Reich shocking, yet still maintained its own system of apartheid, a contradiction that Marable
insists "was made perfectly clear to all." In 1949, actor, singer,

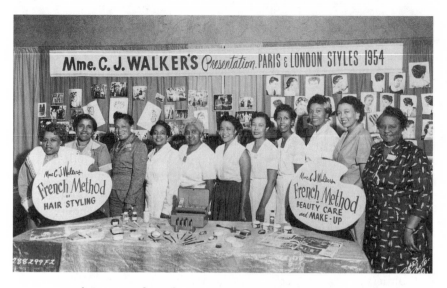

On their return from the 1954 trip to Paris and London, beauticians from Madame C. J. Walker Beauty College presented the French method of hairstyling to a Chicago audience. Courtesy of Vivian G. Harsh, Collection of Afro-American History and Literature, Carter G. Woodson Regional Library, Chicago, Ill., Marjorie Stewart Joyner Collection.

and activist Paul Robeson shamed the United States in a controversial address in Paris when he compared the U.S. policies toward Africa with those of "Hitler and Goebbels."[32] At a time when the United States attempted to project its image as world leader, such international civil rights tactics would prove significant. Thus it was no coincidence that Joyner looked to Europe as a way to reveal the hypocrisy surrounding one of America's fastest growing industries. At best, she found that white-owned beauty schools continued to only take "one or two black girls" on a token basis as they did her, "but not men." Repeatedly Joyner was told "We can't have black students here [because] they'll run our white students away," harkening back to long-held fears of the intermingling of white women and black men. According to Joyner you had to be imaginative, "And you had to think up ways, and things, and procedures in order to beat this so-called color line, this Jim Crowism." Since "we couldn't get into white organizations" in this country, Joyner decided in 1954 to take 195 black cosmetology students to Paris and Rome to receive training from those whom the NHCA undoubtedly embraced as the "masters of the trade." Ironically, then, Joyner used the white hairdressing industry's own Eurocentric definition of professionalism to challenge their credibility. The students who traveled to Europe with Joyner not only made "front page news." But it was also the first time such a large group of professional black women traveled abroad, and their European hosts treated them with an unprecedented degree of respect, dining, for example, with the Duke and Duchess of Windsor aboard the S.S. United States and attending Paris' Moulin Rouge night club where they met the famous Josephine Baker.[33]

Besides targeting the industry specifically, beauticians also used their shops during the postwar period to aid their communities and to form information networks to fight for social

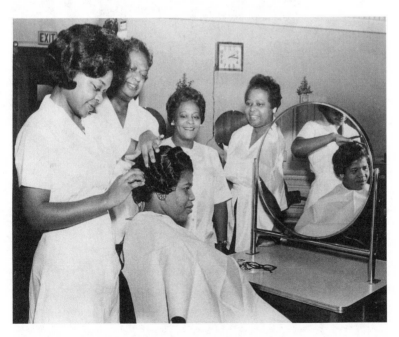

Hairstyling demonstration at beauty shops competition, Chicago, c. 1940s. Courtesy of Vivian G. Harsh, Collection of Afro-American History and Literature, Carter G. Woodson Regional Library, Chicago, Ill., Marjorie Stewart Joyner Collection.

"Growing Faster Than the Dark Roots on a Platinum Blonde"

change and equality. On the one hand, this meant using their hairdressing skills for charity. In 1950, the NHCA was encouraging a "welfare project" after hearing about a United Press story entitled "Hair-Do Aids Mentally Ill." Apparently, beauticians, in association with the "Baltimore hairdressers organization," were offering free haircuts and permanents to patients at

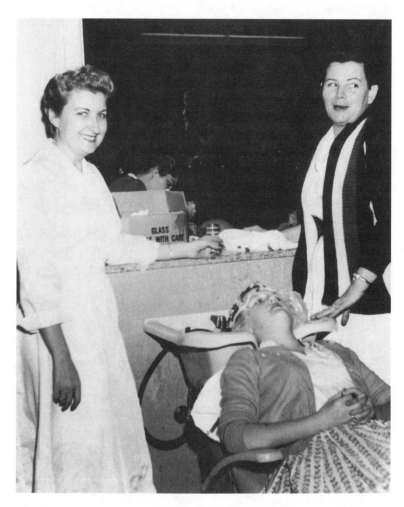

Permanents given to underprivileged children for National Beauty Salon Week, 1957. Courtesy of the Southwest Collection, Texas Tech University, Texas Association of Accredited Beauty Culturists.

"Growing Faster Than the Dark Roots on a Platinum Blonde"

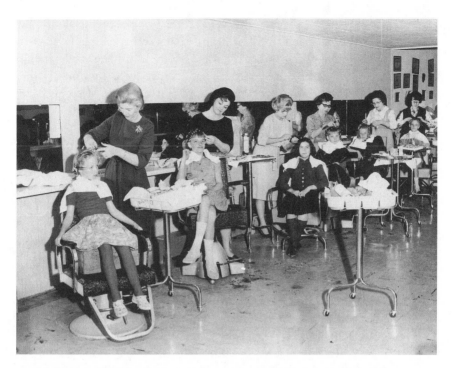

Needy children of Brownwood, Texas, elementary schools, 1964. Courtesy of the Southwest Collection, Texas Tech University, Texas Association of Accredited Beauty Culturists.

the State Hospital at Crownsville, Maryland. Dr. Jacob Morgenstern, who worked with the Baltimore beauticians, claimed that "Many times here in our hospital I have seen the beauty treatment mark the road back for some mentally Ill person." Thus the NHCA, along with countless numbers of local organizations, encouraged similar charity work across the country.[34] On the other hand, the postwar period saw African-American hairdressers continuing the fight for civil rights. Ella Martin, who started the Poro Beauty College in Atlanta and the Georgia Beauty Culturists League, was involved in volunteer work and voter registration drives. Beauty shops, Martin explained, were used "to get them [her customers] interested in voting and to . . . educate them to go to the polls to vote."[35] Bernice Robinson's political activism also "turned her Charleston beauty shop into a political outpost." "In 1951 or '52," Robinson recalled, "Joe Brown took over the NAACP, and that's when we really started making something of the Charleston branch." The membership increased "from three hundred to way over a thousand" and sometimes she was "working so hard getting people to register to vote that I would leave people under the dryer to take others down to the registration office to get them registered."[36]

The beauty shop's role in the Civil Rights Movement, in part, reflected its importance to the community's life. But it was also about economic independence. In the mid-1940s, Myles Horton, who organized and directed the Highlander Folk School (HFS) in Monteagle, Tennessee, which was designed to bring blacks and whites together to challenge segregation, explained the importance of beauty operators in the fight for civil rights. According to Horton, "what you had to do in the pre-civil rights period was to find black people who for the most part were in situations where they weren't too dependent on white people. Otherwise, they would lose their jobs for coming." And it was for that reason, Aldon Morris argues, that the Civil Rights Movement attracted black ministers, funeral home directors, union members, independent small farmers, and, of course, beauticians. Horton found that beauticians were respected not only because they were entrepreneurs, "small businesswomen, you know," but "they were usually better educated than other people, and most of all they were independent. They were independent of white control." It was in Horton's words "sheer accident" that he noticed that "some of the people that came to Highlander were beauticians." And it was this connection between independence and beauty shops that inspired Horton to run workshops at Highlander "just for beauticians." Organizing beauticians raised few suspicions, since most people assumed that Horton's interests were strictly vocational. "They thought that I was bringing these beauticians together to talk about straightening hair or whatever the hell they do." Instead, "I was just using them because they were community leaders and they were independent," which is why Horton "used to use beauticians' shops all over the South to distribute Highlander literature on integration."[37]

As Horton's experience makes clear, the beauty shop's contribution to the Civil Rights Movement reflected its status as a kind of "halfway house." Unlike the church and other prominent institutions, the beauty shop was a less visible institution, which allowed it to more readily challenge the racial status quo without the added pressure more prominent institutions faced. In particular, the beauty shop was less visible to whites. The predominance of the small neighborhood shop, its one or two operators, and an informal atmosphere ensured that hairdressing would remain associated with the home and domesticity, despite the number of different roles beauticians and their shops played. Moreover, because the beauty parlor was generally identified as female space, men, like Myles Horton, paid little attention to its day-to-day activity. Unlike the church, Aldon Morris argues, "halfway houses" were less visible and lacked "broad support and a visible platform," while providing invaluable resources such as "skilled activists, tactical knowledge, media contacts, workshops, knowledge of past movements, and a vision of a future society," qualities found in many beauty shops.[38]

Whether or not beauty operators used their shops to support the war or to fight for civil rights, after World War II a visit to the beauty shop had become part of a woman's routine. In 1948, a survey of beauty shop attendance revealed that 35.7 percent of the women surveyed frequented beauty shops. One year later, the figure had climbed to 40.9 percent. In 1950, it was 44.7 percent and by 1953, over half (52 percent) indicated that they went to beauty shops to have their hair done.[39] A survey in *Vogue* supported those findings and showed that the average reader visited the beauty salon every two weeks while nearly a quarter (385 of 1,779) went once a week.[40] In the 1950s, beauty shops also began to enjoy the regularity of the "standing appointment." In Chicago, shop owner Jack H. Goldberg "doesn't have to worry much about tomorrow's business," because his customers keep "standing appointments once a week or once every two weeks."[41] Indicative of their popularity, the number of shops had also been increasing dramatically since the Depression. In 1938, there were 40,000 shops up from 5,000 in 1900. By 1953, there were 135,000 beauty shops and the vast majority were owner-operator shops in the "small business" category.[42] Despite the increase, the survey also noted that "hairdressing and beauty cultivation has a long way to go to achieve even a portion of its potential."[43]

In order to realize a greater "portion of its potential," the hair-dressing industry, like cosmetic companies, began to target a new teenage clientele. By 1948, *The American Hairdresser* featured shops that catered exclusively to teenagers along with practical tips to capture this newly discovered market. Lillian Blackstone, who owned a beauty salon in Brooklyn, New York, boasted that her "Entire Business Is Teens," something that would have been unheard of a generation earlier. Blackstone, whose clientele was composed primarily of high school and college girls, recommended advertising in school newspapers and through P.T.A. bulletins to attract the young beauty patron. She also publicized her business by offering graduating classes "the chance to win a permanent wave with a hair shaping, shampoo and set." On occasion, she wrote a fashion column in a community newspaper entitled "After Pig-tails, What?" Blackstone also suggested that girls bring in pictures of the style they desired, undoubtedly from an increasing array of new fashion magazines designed specifically with the teenage consumer in mind. In addition, because she felt girls were more likely to experiment with their looks than their mothers, she found it useful to hang "before and after" snapshots on the walls of her salon as well as provide magazines that featured the latest styles.[44]

By the 1950s, teenage girls were spending unprecedented amounts of money on hairstyles, cosmetics, and clothes. Elaine Budd, beauty editor of *Seventeen Magazine*, noted that teenagers were not only "8,000,000 strong" but spending four billion dollars of their own money.[45] According to Beth Bailey, dating and consumption in the postwar period meant that boys and girls were increasingly spending money not only on the date but on what was worn and hence purchased before the date. Going steady, Bailey contends, meant attending all school social events, including the prom, which involved the greatest investment in everything from corsages to shoes and dresses and of course hair and make up.[46] Budd, for example, informed salon owners that "hairstyles are of top interest," and hence displays and promotions should center around special events like "graduation, proms, and other big events," including back-to-school specials. Teenagers were, however, a finicky bunch. While some brought their mothers to the shop and further enhanced business, others were reluctant to enter shops they associated with an older crowd. Thus Budd suggested that certain times be set aside especially for teen patronage and instead of tea and coffee have cokes on hand for thirsty customers. She also urged hiring a young operator or beauty consultant because "teenagers find it easier to discuss their problems with and confide their wishes in someone close to their own age," reaffirming the role of the beautician as confidant and suggesting that teenage conversations were as likely to revolve around the problems and concerns surrounding dating and boys as personal looks and style.[47]

Indeed, for many young women the senior prom was not only popular because of the pomp and circumstance; it also meant the special attention they received from the beautician. Like planning a wedding or searching for that perfect dress, frequenting a beauty shop was often a special kind of experience as memorable as the event itself. In her autobiography, *Coming of Age in Mississippi*, Anne Moody describes the events leading up to her high school prom, an event which included a trip to the hairdresser. According to Moody, it was an occasion that allowed her to transcend, at least temporarily, the racism and discrimination that characterized her childhood. On the day she was crowned homecoming queen, Moody recalled that the beautician "pampered" her like a "princess." "Going to the hairdresser made the day seem even more special," especially "since I had gone there only once before in my life."[48]

Of course adult women still composed a significant percentage of beauty shop patronage, a trend that cut across race and class lines. During the 1940s and '50s, African-American women became an increasingly urban population and found new opportunities beyond agriculture and domestic service. With the war's end, black women, reluctant to return to white households, began to enjoy a greater share of jobs not only in manufacturing, but also in clerical and sales work where their numbers increased eightfold. By 1950, the gap between black and white incomes narrowed. Blacks made 41 percent of what whites earned in 1939 and 60 percent in 1950.[49] In the 1940s, market research also revealed that African Americans were the largest consumers of cosmetics and toiletries, a figure that undoubtedly included hair preparations.[50] By 1950, the number of white female wage earners was nearly 30 percent, a trend that would continue especially since "keeping up with the Joneses" increasingly meant having a two-income household. Most wage-earning women, of course, did not regain the relatively high paying jobs in manufacturing that they found during the war. Instead, they worked disproportionately in the service sector, or in the "types of occupations," where, as the Women's Bureau pointed out, "appearance and good grooming are important."[51]

Across the nation, favorable business trends in the beauty-culture industry would continue throughout the 1950s and 1960s. In 1962, *Pageant* magazine declared that "the sky-rocketing business is growing faster than the dark roots on a platinum blonde."[52] *Time* emphasized that the industry's growth was connected to the general upward trend of the nation's economy, which allowed more women to spend money on beauty aids, and because "a woman will give up food before her pursuit of beauty." To support its claims, *Time* turned to statistical evidence. In 1957, the United States spent an estimated $4 billion on beauty supplies and services, which included $1.4 billion in sales on toilet preparations, up 8.3 percent from the previous year. In 1958, the beauty industry predicted its best year yet. Max Factor, president of one of the top five U.S. cosmetic companies, insisted that "a woman who doesn't wear lipstick feels undressed in public." "Unless," he added, "she works on a farm." Because of this attitude, he claimed, "95% of all women over the age of twelve now use at least one of the products manufactured by the U.S. beauty industry." Hair coloring, "hardly respectable a few years ago," quickly became a $35 million "do-it-yourself" industry while contributing $200 million to the beauty shop industry. According to *Time*, three out of ten women either "tint, rinse, or bleach their hair."[53] In 1958, the United States Census reported that there were 110,000 beauty parlors across the nation, which *Pageant* magazine claimed "lightened the purses of beauty-bound females to the tune of $1 billion, more than double the 1954 total." In 1961, *The American Hairdresser* reported that nearly three billion was spent in 150,000 salons, 90 percent on hairstyling, while the remaining 10 percent was spent on facials, manicures, and various other services, further evidence that "the country has lost its head over hair."[54]

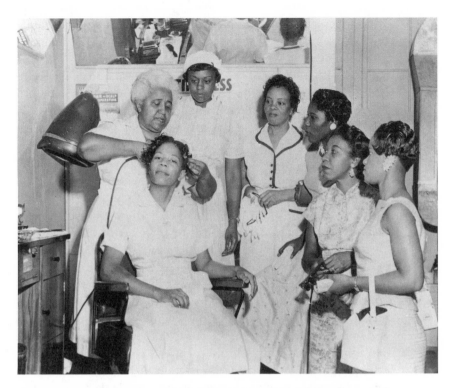

Marjorie Stewart Joyner demonstrating "Satin Tress," a new hair relaxer prod-
uct, 1949. Courtesy of Vivian G. Harsh, Collection of Afro-American History and
Literature, Carter G. Woodson Regional Library, Chicago, Ill., Marjorie Stewart
Joyner Collection.

While the number of hairdressing salons dramatically increased, so too did a wide range of do-it-yourself products. In
the 1950s, magazines like *Ebony* were filled with advertisements
for items like the "Silky Straight Home Beauty Kit," for only
$2.24 plus tax, which was designed for all types of hair—"fine,
coarse, hard-to-manage and normal." Some of these magazines
also featured "Perma-Strate—The Original Cold Permanent Hair
Straightener," which came with an endorsement from stars like
Sarah Vaughan, Dizzy Gillespie, Louis Jordan, Dinah Washington, Count Basie, Isabelle Cooley, and Erskine Hawkins and which
read "These Stars Agree!" Perma-Strate for "Natural Looking
Straight Hair." Wigs and switches were also being advertised

with prices that ranged from three to thirty dollars and a guarantee to achieve the long sweeping "Page Boy" look. Other popular items included marcel irons, straightening combs, and small "oil stoves" with wicks sold separately. While individuals undoubtedly bought such items for personal use, entrepreneurs just starting up could also buy these products and, with some skill, offer beauty services with little investment.[55]

Many do-it-yourself products created concerns for hairdressers. The "cold wave," a chemical means of curling hair, made its debut in the late 1940s and caused many shop owners to worry about their businesses. The "Home Permanent," *The American Hairdresser* declared, "Must Be Eliminated." Home permanent kits, many feared, would not only lead to a decline in the number of customers but could ultimately undermine the price structure because shop employees could, if they so desired, offer cold waving as a private enterprise at a price lower than what the shop could afford. Just like hair straighteners and other solutions, home permanents did attract a considerable amount of consumer interest, and some women even achieved the look they wanted without the extra time and money typically spent at a beauty shop.[56]

But even the most simple do-it-yourself jobs could turn into disasters. Lillian Blackstone did not seem particularly concerned that there were "a certain few who like to try something on their own, like those who cut their own bangs." Not to worry, insisted Blackstone, "eventually they came crying to me to right the wrong they have done."[57] In fact, when women had the tools, it seemed that few had the skills to achieve the look they wanted. Postwar hair styles also remained too intricate, and a good perm demanded both skill and patience. In 1958, *Time* magazine declared that Toni home permanents "temporarily threatened to empty the beauty shops," but the "poodle," which "consists of chopping off a woman's hair to about three inches and then twisting the surviving strands into a hundred or so corkscrews," filled the beauty parlors up again. Indeed, home-permanent sales dropped nearly 30 percent a year after they were introduced.[58] It seems that "too many housewives with one eye on the children and the other on dinner botched the whole thing."[59]

While do-it-yourself perms created an annoyance for beauty shop owners, the relative scarcity of operators created the gravest

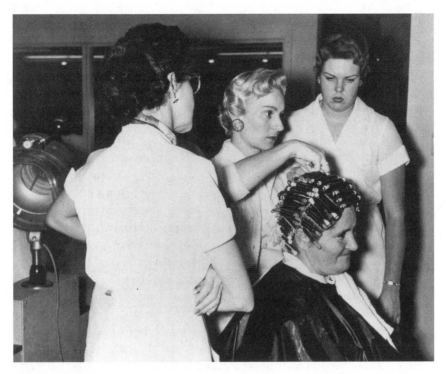

Perming hair, 1957. Courtesy of the Southwest Collection, Texas Tech University, Texas Association of Accredited Beauty Culturists.

concerns for industry leaders. During the postwar period, the hairdressing industry enjoyed unprecedented economic growth. Yet *The American Hairdresser* compared the labor shortage of the early 1950s to the crisis of the war years. In 1950, for example, the census revealed that the number of women employed in beauty service had dropped 8 percent since 1940. According to the Women's Bureau, the decrease in the number of female operators may have reflected the difficulty some women found in gaining access to training since many cosmetology classes, especially in public vocational schools, were filled with men. Approximately 37,000 male veterans trained as hairdressers under the GI Bill of Rights, although few of these men turned to hairdressing as a permanent occupation because of the relative abundance of good paying jobs.[60] Instead, industry leaders blamed the shortage on women because they left the profession shortly after marriage. Herbert Rosen, vice president of Helene Curtis Sales, insisted that women worked on average only four to five years in the trade because they "have a habit of getting a husband and then acquiring some children." Although in 1950 the Women's Bureau reported that half of all operators were married, Rosen complained that "this process [marriage] takes them out of the shop and into the home." Ironically, then, the labor shortage that now plagued the industry in part reflected years of reform efforts on the part of the NHCA designed to separate beauty shops from the domestic sphere and dissuade married women from setting up the kind of shops that best fit the demands family life made.[61]

In 1952, beauty school enrollments continued to decline and industry leaders began to voice their concerns, again harkening back to the difficulties they faced during the war. The NHCA insisted that the industry was facing a "grave" crisis as beauty schools continued to report "serious drops in enrollment." According to the NHCA, "convincing young men and women beauty work is a worthwhile career, cannot be left solely to the schools." Instead, the NHCA, insisted, "It is a job for everyone." *The American Hairdresser* urged shop owners to take action, learn the names of every high school in their community, and promote the adoption of vocational courses in beauty culture. Some shop owners were even willing to sponsor a student's education, paying her or his way through beauty school in exchange for a three-year commitment to the salon owner.[62] Robert R. Hoffman, Revlon Products sales manager, feared the labor shortage would resurrect old problems associated with the war, when the shortage of operators was so severe that "many shops were forced to close" or operate on "a curtailed basis because the number of operators was extremely limited." Not only did "Mrs. Consumer" find it a "chore" to make an appointment, but Hoffman insisted that the quality of work was substandard and that the service given to patrons was often "discourteous."[63]

One way to handle the labor shortage was to get more out of each operator. Thus *The American Hairdresser* presented a series of time and motion studies to reduce costs. Through pictures and words an "expert" revealed ways to reduce the time needed to complete the most complicated hair styles. "One of the most flagrant wastes in Time and Motion in the beauty shop is in the actual performance of services," insisted "expert" Robert Fiance. Even if the operators "produce a good final result," the methods used were not necessarily the most efficient. According to Fiance, "we do not even realize where we are losing time and wasting energy or that there might be a quicker, better method of performing the same services." Thus Fiance explained in detail the most effective way to hold the scissors, hair, and comb between one's fingers as well as the exact number of rollers each head of hair needed to reach the optimum amount of curl. While too few rollers could leave a customer dissatisfied, too many were inefficient—a waste of time and money.[64] Above all, "the operator must understand that in the creation of a hairdo, he or she is essentially acting the part of an engineer." The hairdresser, who Fiance defined in masculine terms, "is literally building something with material (hair)."[65]

The time and motion studies Fiance advocated directly reflected the ongoing tension between professionalism and the kind of beauty shop culture neighborhood owners and operators desired. An emphasis on speed, for example, threatened the relationships between customers and operators, relationships that remained crucial in negotiating a favorable work culture. Robert Hoffman warned that the labor shortage gave an unfair advantage to the operator. A diminishing surplus labor pool meant in Hoffman's mind that "anyone who had an operator or two didn't dare to insist on better work or more courteous service." In particular, Hoffman found that current conditions allowed operators to refuse any task they found displeasing. "Operators who previously would pitch in and do a manicure, an eyebrow job or facial or scalp treatment," he complained, "refused to do this work." Instead, they chose to labor exclusively as hairdressers, engaging only in "the big-four: . . . permanent waving, hair cuts, coloring, and styling."[66]

In addition, time and motion studies were the result of new consumer demands for styles that required far greater degrees of time, skill, and finesse, further reasserting the hairdresser's skill and worker control. By the early 1950s, the "poodle" hair cut seemed well suited for young and old alike, especially since there were dozens of variations all named appropriately enough after the other members of the canine family.[67] The poodle, however, required constant attention, including a haircut every two weeks, a frequent permanent wave for women with naturally straight hair, and typically 125 curlers. Yet, the high maintenance do only seemed to attract beauty parlor patrons. In fact, some shops reported "poodling hundreds of heads a day." By the 1950s and early 1960s, bouffants and beehives were all the rage which meant hairdressers would spend even more time with each client to produce a look that some described as everything from "cotton candy" to a "haystack swept back from the forehead and swelling dangerously from the crown."[68] Transforming straight, stringy hair into gravity defying hairstyles required extensive amounts of back combing and teasing, not to mention enormous quantities of hairspray. As well, curly hair usually had to be straightened first, then curled and combed into place. Dorothy Williams, a Missouri woman, remembered when bouffants were all the rage in the 1950s, it was "one of the busiest times for hairdressers, due to the fact that women couldn't fix this particular style very well by themselves." But she admits it was also the "most difficult style for hairdressers."[69] Lucy Giambusi, who started her beauty shop in 1950 on Philadelphia's South Side, also recalled the connection between the growth of the industry and changes in style. According to Giambusi, women in the 1950s wore what she called the "upsweep," which contrasted sharply with styles from the 1990s where women "wear their hair real stringy [and] long." "Today," Giambusi explained, women "don't even go to the hairdresser that's why the hairdressers are all starving."[70] "Formalized hair-setting practices," then, demanded skill and patience as well as a vast array of "setting lotions, pins or rollers, and dryers." Such styles required trips to the beauty shop not only to have the hair styled, but also to have the hair combed out and washed, something which also took a considerable amount of time and patience. As a result of the latest fashion craze, customers who in years past might have visited a beauty parlor every few months for a permanent wave, now made a trip to the hairdresser's a weekly routine. And just when customers learned one style, new styles demanding new techniques filled the pages of fashion magazines and kept the beauty-conscious woman at her hairdresser's beck and call.[71]

"Growing Faster Than the Dark Roots on a Platinum Blonde"

While these new styles emphasized women's dependency on
their hairdresser's hands, the emphasis on style also elevated
the relative position of male hairdressers in popular culture—a
trend that would only continue in decades to come. Male hairdressers had long been considered professionals, but this new
postwar emphasis on hair transformed male hairdressers from
professionals to pop icons. By the 1960s, Jackie Kennedy's hairdressers, Mr. Kenneth and George Masters, whose work was
featured in *Life* magazine, became as famous as the women who
wore their creations. Indeed, the hairdresser had become, in the
words of one fashion report, an "international celebrity."[72] Like
clothing designers, their new styles filled the pages of fashion
magazines and seemed to change with the season. At a 1961 San
Francisco fall beauty show, "the Pixie, the Beehive, and the
Bubble were out." Instead, "The Airlift," a "stream-lined, up-
swept, puffy hair-do," requiring a gadget called a "poofer," was
all the craze.[73] By 1962, some of Masters' more famous coiffures
included the "Little European Boy," the "Cyclone Cut," "The
Snob," and "The Killer Cut." And regardless of whether it was
Jackie Kennedy or the girl next door, hairstylist Robert
Williams explained that each new style only made women more
dependent upon the hairdresser's hands. Even when the wind-
blown "Italian cut" became popular, "[W]omen soon discovered that it was more painstaking to look causal than pin-
curled" and "found they no longer could set their hair themselves" because, Williams noted, they "didn't know how to use
rollers or the techniques of back combing."[74]

The popularity of elaborate and everchanging styles also affected the neighborhood beauty shop in many different ways.
First, it meant that the beauty ritual became part of larger numbers of women's lives. Not only had the number of shops more
than tripled since the mid-1930s, but more working- and middle-
class women were likely to attend their favorite beauty shop—
usually a small owner-operator business—on a weekly basis. As
a result, postwar customers and hairdressers alike generally
identified the beauty parlor with all the things the NHCA had
for so long been trying to eliminate: the informal atmosphere,
the "unprofessional" chit chat and gossip, and the causal mixing of domestic duties with business, all of which reinforced a

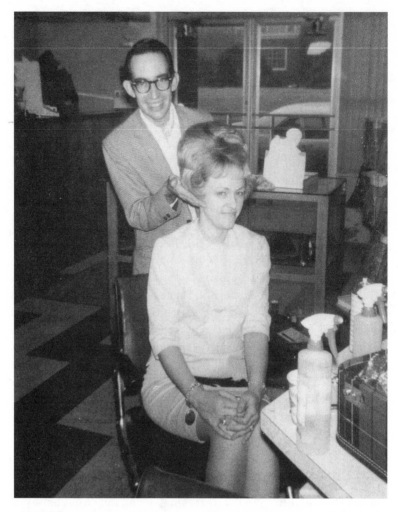

The bouffant—thanks to the hairdresser's hands, 1968. Courtesy of the Southwest Collection, Texas Tech University, Texas Association of Accredited Beauty Culturists.

pink-collar professionalism that even the NHCA seemed willing to embrace.

Indeed, because the changes in style required a considerable amount of time and frequent if not weekly visits to the beauty shop, women found that the beauty shop had become an important ritual, making the neighborhood beauty operator more than

Washington, D.C., like many African-American women, worked as a domestic laborer and decided to attend beauty school at night. Her training allowed her to eventually open her own business, Alice's Beauty Salon, which she described as being open virtually around the clock. "We did not have closing hours then. We took as many as four customers, as early as six o'clock a.m., before they went to work, and as many as ten in the evening after work." In fact, the doors of her business never really closed because she also cared for her customers day and night—mentally and physically. Her thirty-six years as a beauty operator taught her that "beauticians have to be more than hairdressers." While they may earn their money dressing hair, they were also required to be "doctors, advisors, good listeners, relaxation therapists and more." In other words, the hairdresser was someone to trust and rely on no matter what kind of problem the patron was facing. According to Murray, beauticians helped women who needed to escape the everyday pressures of home, job, and family. "Often, when women are upset at home," she found, "they will either go shopping or to the hair parlor seeking relief." But concern for a customer's welfare, she insisted, did not stop at her shop's front door. Sometimes she made sure customers made it to their homes safely. Indeed, "being there" for one's customer involved "a wide range of services," because in Murray's words, she was "always concerned about [the] customers' well-being," a concern that created intimate bonds between the beauty operator and her customers, and one that an increasing number of women shared.[75]

During the 1950s, the NHCA recognized and reaffirmed the beauty shop's importance to women's everyday lives and the beauty shop's link to domesticity. The beauty shop, the NHCA now realized, had to create an atmosphere amenable to the needs of mothers and their children, something operators long argued was necessary for business success. Thus *The American Hairdresser* featured a new kind of shop as its model, one in which the male expert was conspicuously absent. The journal praised Maggie's Shop located in Culver City, California, because of its clever layout designed to accommodate children. While evening appointments were available, Maggie's Shop offered a play yard with a sandpile "where tots may be left to play with complete safety while mother had her hair done" during the day. Maggie also carefully chose "unbreakable" toys and, of course, provided "supervision at all times."[76] *The American Hairdresser* also suggested that shop owners provide "comic books and children's magazines to keep little hands and minds busy . . . [or] provide little favors like chewing gum and candy if the child is good." And if any of the operators had some free time, they might try brushing the child's hair. The journal also thought of another "clever trick" in which the beauty operator could give the child a magnet and be sent around the shop floor to scavenge "stray hairpins," making better use of the child's energy as well as the operator's patience.[77] Most important of all, the NHCA praised the neighborhood salon because it "created a friendly, informal relationship between salon and patron," an ideology the NHCA now understood as "a potential business builder."[78] Thus unlike the 1930s when the NHCA castigated shop owners when children were present and when women chatted away the day, by the 1950s, it praised the efficiency of the beauty shop where children crawled under the hairdresser's feet in search of stray hairpins.

The postwar labor shortage also meant new opportunities for women at a time when they were increasingly identified with the domestic sphere. Nearly half (four out of ten) of all beauty operators were in business for themselves in the 1950s, and that number undoubtedly overlooked the thousands of beauty shops tucked away in women's homes. Indeed, most states did not prohibit home shops, and, as mentioned previously, national hairdressing organizations were even encouraging the kind of shop that they had for so long condemned.[79] By allowing women to supplement the family income with a clientele based primarily on their neighbors and other familiar faces, small owner-operator beauty shops flourished alongside the more cosmopolitan salons that were found in the most fashionable shopping areas of America's towns and cities. Above all, women were challenging the 1950s myth perpetuated by men like George Gallup and Evan Hill, who conducted a survey of 2,300 women and found that the American woman was uninterested in either business or politics. In beauty shops an unprecedented number of women were not only owning and operating their own shops instead of dedicating themselves full time to their homes and their husbands and families, but also managing employees, negotiating business deals with other entrepreneurs, overseeing inventories, and cultivating and maintaining a clientele.[80]

The labor shortage also meant better wages. In 1949, the average weekly earnings for a beautician was just over twenty-seven dollars. By the 1950s, most beauticians were experiencing an increase in their weekly earnings. According to the Women's Bureau in 1950, new beauty operators usually "began at a relatively low salary, depending on locality and type of shop." But in a year or two the operator could easily "double her earnings by building up her clientele." For example, a midwestern state reported that earnings for the "average beautician were $35 to $50 weekly in 1950." Four years later beauticians with less than one year of experience earned $50 to $60 per week," and "experienced operators made from $75 to $100 per week," not including tips. And in exclusive salons, hairdressers could earn more than a $150 a week.[81] By comparison, the average wage for waitresses nationwide was three dollars a day in 1953.[82]

The relatively high wages beauticians earned meant some women were able to redefine their stereotypical role within the context of the family economy. In the 1940s, Virginia Martell began attending a beauty school that cost her $125. Martell attended beauty school each morning, while her husband watched their newborn baby. When she returned from school, he went to work, and she "would do all the diapers which [she] had soaked the day before." Martell recalled that "between doing diapers and steaming bottles, and taking care of the baby, I would try to study very hard because I couldn't fail." Martell's hard work paid off for she graduated with "an 88 average" and "set up a little shop for [her] neighbors." For a "dollar or two dollars" she would give a haircut, a permanent, or a shampoo and set to "make some extra money." No sooner had she opened her shop when her husband was "taken into the service." While he was gone, Martell explained the "government allowed me $100 per month." By the time her husband returned from the service, her son was two years old, and she had saved $1,000 with the help of her beauty shop earnings. For the next few years, Martell continued to work as a beautician and continued to save her earnings. Several times the family moved and each time they had to settle for a basement apartment until she had saved $3,500, again with the help of her beauty shop.[83]

In fact, with relatively few independently-owned businesses, beauty shops, no matter how meager, often provided the basis for an entire community's post-war economic expansion. During the 1940s, Foster's Beauty Salon owned by Hazel Foster of Tippah County, Mississippi, primarily offered "pressing and curling" to an African-American clientele. The services combined brought in less than seventy cents per customer. "A press was $.25, and it cost $.35 for a thermal curl." Moreover, it was labor intensive. "We didn't even have hot water then. We would heat water on a hot plate, and recline the client in a big bowl of warm water to wash her hair." Yet despite her humble beginnings, her small shop eventually grew into an impressive enterprise that offered a variety of hairstyles, cuts, facials, and even nail services. As her shop grew, so did her role in the community. Not only was Hazel Foster "the first person in Tippah County [Mississippi] to own a telephone in the early '40s," which meant she played a decisive role in her community's life because she "used to run messages around for the neighborhood," but her business eventually included "a motel, day care center, laundromat, funeral home, dormitory for the beauty college and a barber college." Perhaps most significant of all, her salon as of 1988 was still "the only black-owned business in Sherman, Mississippi."[84]

As the experiences of these operators suggest, the neighborhood shop's role in the community changed very little in terms of the community services and personal interaction it had long offered women. But the expansion of the industry meant that the neighborhood shop's services had became a part of the day-to-day lives of an increasing number of women who a generation earlier had never frequented the beauty parlor on such a regular basis. Whether straightened or curled, intricate hair styles not only fueled the growth of an industry, but also created the time and space women as customers and as workers needed to reflect upon and negotiate family and community roles. In fact, as Lulline Long understood, beauty culture was a means to financial success as well as a way to keep youth on the straight and narrow. Whether a beauty shop was simply a place were women could be pampered or a place where female conversations and company helped sort out the problems at hand, the beauty shop had long established its community role in women's lives at a time when the dominant discourse insisted that women remain complacent and domestic bound.

Beginning with World War II and continuing throughout the 1950s and 1960s, the hairdressing industry's economic growth also encouraged a shift in the definition of professionalism. Unlike the preceding decades, when industry leaders derided the neighborhood shop as the bane of the industry, by the 1940s and 1950s, the home shop had become an acceptable model for the industry. On the one hand, the shortage of available women along with the demands of World War II helped legitimize this shift as industry leaders found themselves scrambling to find anyone willing to set up a beauty parlor. On the other hand, this redefinition reflected changes in style and consumer demand. Throughout the period more elaborate dos began to outpace the simple bob, ensuring more entrepreneurial opportunities for women eager to own their own shops and that the neighborhood shop, along with its informal setting and casual talk, would become part of the beauty regime of millions of American women.

At the same time, the growth and challenges that characterized the hairdressing industry in the 1940s and 1950s revealed the degree to which hairdressing associations such as the NHCA were reluctant to cross racial barriers, barriers that had provided structure to the industry throughout the early twentieth century. Even in the face of a labor shortage, when the NHCA willingly recasts its understanding of professionalism to include the female-dominated neighborhood shop, race remained an impenetrable boundary, reinforcing the degree to which professionalism was race based. By the 1960s, those racial barriers appeared as impenetrable as ever. But as the Black Liberation Movement became more visible in the 1960s and 1970s, white corporate America began to look more closely at the profit potential in the black hair-care market. Ultimately, this created a new challenge for African-American and Euro-American hairdressers who found corporate desires attempting to undermine their work culture and independence. This struggle was not only dramatically played out in the context of beauty salons as female operators, white and black, fought to maintain control over their work and professional identities but also across America as changes in style became identified with the political unrest of the 1960s and 1970s.

5

Afros, Cornrows, and Jesus Hair

Corporate America, the Ethnic Market, and the Struggle over Professionalism

One widespread theory on the reason God gave black people our hair in the first place is that God always wanted us to have some business of our very own. God is all-Knowing. God must have foreseen that black people would have less than a head start in the world trade market such as it is currently constructed. So, in another moment of brilliance, God was God. And black hair was black hair.

Ralph Wiley
Why Black People Tend to Shout: Cold Facts
and Wry Views from a Black Man's World

In 1973, nationally syndicated columnist Carl Rowan declared that he had grown disillusioned with the American political scene and "dismayed" to find his readership more interested in "black hair styles" than "real" issues: "what a sad commentary that people should be more concerned about 'afros' and 'corn-rows' than about Vietnam, or the Watergate scandal, or hunger in America, or the drift toward a police state!" Rowan's disappointment came after he had written a column about contemporary African-American hair styles and received hundreds of letters in response to his editorial, far more attention, he admitted, than any of his columns had previously received. Yet he was pleasantly surprised to find that the vast majority of his readers agreed that the "afro" was indeed just a "shortcut to 'pride,'" an obsession that spoke directly to the problems endemic to black America.

With the help of several reassuring letters, Rowan argued that racism would be eliminated only when black youth focused less on the "rhetoric of rage" and instead on "trained intelligence." A junior high school teacher, who had written a letter in response to Rowan, helped clarify his point by suggesting that if "blacks spent as much time in serious learning as they spend on their hair, they could lay the foundation for the greatest civilization." But instead, "these hair styles have reached a mania stage. . . . Pupils will come to class prepared with combs [and] picks, . . . [when] they should have pencils, paper, and related materials."[1]

Despite Rowan's dismissal of the afro as nothing more than a diversion from the real issues at stake, hair styles provide crucial insight into the development of African-American culture from the 1960s to the 1990s and to the response of many African Americans to the end of the Civil Rights and Black Power Movements. But debates over the afro and other hairstyles also shed light on the broader changes in American society since the 1960s. While the tensions surrounding civil rights, gay liberation, black power, and the war in Vietnam translated into violent conflict on city streets across the country, these same tensions were played out through fashion and style as men and women, amidst profound social and cultural change, were attempting to come to terms with their own identity and understanding of race, class, and gender. For many Americans, then, hair became the symbol of political rebellion, and changes in style stood as a rejection of conservative politics, corporate images of respectability, bourgeois esthetics, and conventional definitions of beauty.

The social changes that characterized America in the 1960s and 1970s were also equally divisive within the context of the hairdressing industry itself. In the 1970s, corporate America not only strived to reorganize the basic structure of the industry with the introduction of unisex chain salons, but also attempted to exploit, control, and manipulate the "ethnic market." Both trends profoundly shaped the beauty salon's work culture as well as hairstylists' own understanding of work, skill, and professionalism. Although the industry had long been divided along lines of race, class, and gender, the politics of hair brought these tensions to the surface and exposed the contradictions in the industry as it tried to rationalize, routinize, and homogenize the labor process.

Changes in the hairdressing industry also reflect the broader debates over hair that polarized Americans across the country. Corporate America's interest in unisex salons and the "ethnic market" developed around the debates over changing hair styles. But corporate America failed to understand the complexity of the issues involved. While beauty shops fostered vibrant women's cultures, these cultures grew out of racial segregation. The introduction of chain salons and attempts to "court the ethnic market" threatened the boundaries around which the beauty shop and the hairstylists' position in the industry had developed. In short, industry leaders tried to break down racial, class, and gender boundaries in their pursuit of larger profits. But hairstylists responded to these changes in unexpected ways. Changes in the industry affected the work culture of the salon and stylists' struggles to maintain control over the shop floor, struggles which limited the extent to which the industry has changed and the degree to which corporate America monopolized the "ethnic market."

In 1965, columnist Russell Baker asserted that "A man's right to wear his hair as he wants to is one of the glories of a free society, and one of the first actions of tyrants is invariably to groom their subject males in a uniform haircut." Throughout the twentieth century, he argued, "Prisons, drill-sergeants, Nazism and the modern organization all have a common goal in their need to suppress individualism. . . . Nazis used the crewcut. The modern business-organization man is marked by the corporate trim—a hint of sideburns, no hair hanging over the collar, [and] no forelocks more than three inches long." Thus Baker encouraged young, white men to fashion a rebellion all their own and grow their hair long.[2] Yet Baker only alluded to part of the inspiration for the new fashion trend. Bill Severn has pointed to rock 'n' roll groups, movies, and musicals that convinced a generation of baby boomers to forgo frequent trips to the barber shop. "Within months after the landing of the Beatles," Severn recalls, "male moptops began a sprout-out and by the spring of 1965 the American crew cut was dying if not dead." By 1968, the musical *Hair* had opened in New York and, with "its fresh music, words, and a hint of nudity," captured the spirit of a young generation who made long hair a symbol of their rebellion.[3] Yet from wherever the inspiration for long hair came, one thing was certain, insisted Edward Miller, an unemployed waiter living in Haight Ashbury in the late 1960s: "It takes a lot of guts to live like you want to [and] Dress like you want to."[4]

The popularity of longer hair was not limited to the rebellious, however. As early as 1967, the *New York Times* reported that "after several years of excoriating pop singers, arty types, and their own teen-age sons, city men of middle age are letting their hair grow." Indeed, long hair was now the "In" look in New York City and even "Such traditional squares as stockbrokers, physicians, and corporation executives are relinquishing the crew cuts to which they have clung since they returned from service in World War II."[5] Bill Severn found that by the 1970s, "in most city high school corridors and on college campuses there was hardly a short-hair in sight." In fact, one school official claimed that "even fathers who come to P.T.A. meetings have long hair."[6]

The trend toward longer hair marked a significant change in the hairdressing industry. In the early 1960s, it seemed that the industry would remain sex segregated. While barber shops offered men "a place to give in to their vanities, talk to other men,— and get a good haircut," neighborhood beauty shops had long been considered a distinctly female sphere.[7] Even in the late 1960s, there were a lot of men who, like automobile salesman Robert Cheatum, would never consider using a beauty shop for men. "You'd never get me in a hair net or under the dryer," insisted Cheatum. Elmer Hoyal, "a tire man," agreed that he "don't go to places like that." In fact, he never went anywhere that needed "a fancy hair cut," just out "to the baseball games . . . Kezar for the 49ers [or] Maybe the wrestling matches," insinuating that a barber shop was all a working-class man needed to look respectable.[8] Francis Smith, a white midwestern woman who worked as a beauty operator in the early 1960s, recalled that "back then we didn't have a lot of men come into the shop. See that was wrong; men didn't do that."[9]

Despite the reluctance of both men and women to cross that gender line, by the early 1970s, "the natural look" had swept from coast to coast, and women were spending less time with their hairdressers than in previous decades, while more men

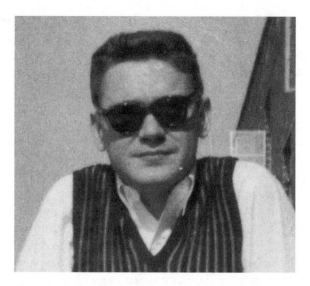

The crew cut, 1956. From the author's collection.

began frequenting beauty shops. In San Francisco, Patty Swig observed the gendered transformation of the hairstyling industry
within the context of her own family. "My father," she declared,
now "goes to my mother's hairdresser. My brother goes to mine.
And my husband's letting his hair grow so he can go, too." She
thought that men increasingly "feel women's stylists know long
hair better," an attitude that not only redefined the character of
the beauty shop, but threatened the very existence of barber
shops.[10]

Barbers had long feared competition with women's hairdressers
and had successfully established laws in many states that forbade
men from patronizing beauty salons. But the battle lines were
drawn more sharply in the late 1960s, with men growing their
hair longer and making fewer trips to the barber shop. On the
East Coast the decline in the number of barber shops was so dramatic, it compelled many barbers to take collective action. In
Perth Amboy, New Jersey, for example, "the haircutting business
is so bad that veteran barbers here have resorted to a tactic they
last used in the great depression of the 1930s." Stephen Fransa,
who had been a barber for fifty years, helped organize a boycott
aimed at any shops in his community that employed long-haired

men, whom he argued were threatening his own livelihood. In just two years his business had declined by 40 percent and approximately five hundred barber shops had closed down throughout the state. "We're blaming those teenagers and some businessmen . . . who haven't had a haircut in a year or so," complained Fransa. A boycott seemed the best solution to many barbers who felt "funny" spending their "good money" in a place where the employees had "long hair."[11] Some barbers, of course, joined the bandwagon and attempted to change their image by calling themselves men's hairstylists. But as one female hairstylist put it, the barber only knows two cuts: "a young man's cut and old man's cut." And a change in name simply ignored the expertise and skill needed to style hair and did little to satisfy a new generation of long-haired customers who were experimenting not only with the length of their hair, but also with color and perms.[12]

As the trend in long hair continued to grow, so too, did the decline in the number of barber shops across the country, especially those that still offered standard crew cuts. The U.S. Census figures reported that between 1972 and 1982 the number of barber shops fell by more than 28 percent.[13] It seemed that "the twirling barber poles, the low rumbling of fellow men's voices, the smell of cigars, and the traditional leather chairs" were nothing more than a childhood memory for a generation of men coming of age in the 1970s.[14]

Barbers were not the only ones upset with the change in men's hairstyles. Despite the growing popularity of long hair, the controversy over men's hair raged on through the early 1970s and was played out in the context of schools, courtrooms, sporting events, and amusement parks while everyone from grade-school boys to fire fighters, taxicab drivers, and professional sports players became entangled in the controversy.[15] At times, the controversy over hair turned deadly. On April 14, 1971, the *San Francisco Chronicle* reported that a "Castro Valley man killed his 20-year-old son after a row about the boy's long hair and [his] 'negative attitude toward society.'"[16] More typically, however, the struggle over long hair was contested through words and heated debates. As early as 1968, advice columnist Ann Landers declared that "hair has become one of the most passionately argued subjects of our time—ranking third after Vietnam and race riots." In 1971,

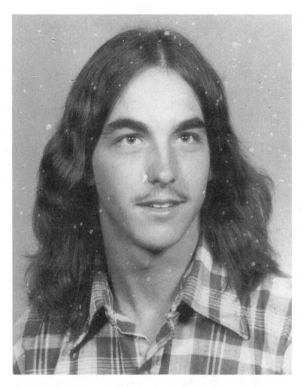

The "Jesus" look, 1973. Courtesy of Morris Fitch.

the issue of hair remained divisive. Writing to Ann Landers, one man was not only fed up with long hair, but specifically with "kids" who attempted to justify their looks by using Jesus as an example: "If one more long-haired hippie tells me Jesus had long hair," he declared, "I will personally kick him in the teeth." The angry reader admitted that "nobody knows what Jesus looked like," but he thought the "best information" is in the "Bible, Corinthians, Chapter 11, Verse 14: 'Does not even nature itself teach you that, if a man have long hair, it is a shame unto him?'" The letter writer thought "Any kid who wants to wear his hair long ought to be man enough to do it without saying he is imitating Jesus."[17]

According to Joshua Freeman, the anger directed towards long-haired men often had class dimensions that reflected concerns over changing definitions of masculinity against the back-

drop of the Vietnam War. Construction workers, for example, insisted that many draft dodgers and anti-war protesters, who were
known for their long hair, had benefitted undeservingly from
their class privilege. Freeman found one tradesman who expressed his frustrations towards anti-war protesters: "here were
these kids, rich kids, who could go to college, who didn't have to
fight, they are telling you your son died in vain. It makes you feel
as though your whole life is shit, just nothing." As well, Freeman
found that at times "pro-war construction workers singled out
anti-war protesters with the longest hair for assault" and shouted
down "special targets" by calling them "faggots." Freeman argues
that long hair symbolized a new masculinity that long-haired
men based on "traditionally female notions [of] sensuality and
sensitivity" and "rejected the idea that manhood meant physical
strength and aggressiveness." But the frequency with which construction workers referred to long-haired men as "faggots" suggests that while class boundaries were being exposed and challenged in the late 1960s and early '70s, so too were the boundaries
defining heterosexuality.[18]

References to effeminacy were, in fact, quite common throughout the 1960s and 1970s when it came to hair. Many contemporaries believed that long hair stood for all that was wrong in
the country, especially with regard to the behavior of young men.
Yet long hair symbolized more than just a generation gap; it
threatened heterosexual definitions of masculinity and as much
as the long-haired man was characterized as a "hippie," "pot-
smoker," or "radical," he was also described as a "homosexual"
and a "freak." Advice columnist Abigail Van Buren insisted quite
simply that "long hair is feminine and short hair is masculine."[19]
Eugene W. Vess of Salem, Virginia, who had been a barber since
1946, not only agreed but thought it was "pitiful" that "you can't
tell the girls from the boys any more." Vess was "sick of looking
at people and wondering what they are" and out of frustration
decided to close down his barber shop.[20] Journalist Joseph Whitney also maintained that the reason "parents are ashamed of long-
haired sons" was primarily because they associated long hair with
"effeminacy, draft-card burning, and beatniks."[21]

Just as long hair created controversy over male sexuality so,
too, did the image of the male hairdresser. George Chauncey ar-

served as metaphors for gay experiences and revealed the way gay men frequently negotiated a double life. "Putting their hair up," Chauncey notes, "meant men kept their gay lives hidden from potentially hostile straight observers," while "dropped hairpins" caught only the attention of other gay men.[22] In a sociological investigation of Chicago hairdressers, David Schroder finds that the influx of immigrant men into traditionally female-dominated occupations such as women's hairdressing often convinced native-born men that the occupation was unmanly and "not the kind of job men were supposed to have."[23] By World War II, male hairdressers were inextricably bound to a gay identity. According to Allan Bérubé, during the war men who worked as beauticians were given specific tasks in the military that "fit popular notions of what it meant to be queer."[24] And whether or not hairdressers were "queer," Schroder insisted many of his interviewees in the 1970s "lisped; talked with high, feminine voices; swished; and handled themselves in a fragile, feminine manner." Moreover, in his words, "it is a well known fact" that in hairdressing there were "freaks of all sorts," including "known homosexuals."[25]

Because hairdressers were often associated with effeminacy and long-haired men were often considered "pot smokers," "homosexuals," and "freaks," the industry set out to change the image of men's hairstyling in order to attract a new male clientele whose masculinity would not be compromised when entering a salon. The easiest way to make men feel comfortable was to mitigate anything remotely feminine and seemingly unprofessional, something that industry leaders long wanted to accomplish. "A lot of salons let men know—by changing their tone of advertising as well as . . . the style of their decor—that male clients were indeed welcome." As a consequence, a more gender neutral, businesslike atmosphere replaced the image of the "pink and frilly 'beauty parlor.'" Terms such as "beauty," for example, began to disappear in favor of more generic names such as "hairstyling salon" and "family hair care center."[26] These new so-called unisex salons, which became part of an increasing number of nationwide chains, transformed the beauty shop ritual into a more business-like atmosphere—all in the name of customer convenience and an expanding market. In fact, in less than a decade, "The pink chairs

[were] gone and with them the old cans of formaldehyde-smelling hair spray, the rubber rollers, the plastic window curtains, and names like Bertha's Temple of Beauty." While traditional beauty shops still flourish in small towns, inner-city neighborhoods, and suburban enclaves, they have dramatically decreased in number in the face of large corporate competition. Between 1975 and 1985, "more than 60,000 'mom and pop' beauty salons and barber shops" had "folded." The publisher of a leading trade journal, *Modern Salon*, believed small shops failed because they could not "cater to people's needs."[27]

Even popular culture seemed intent on altering the image of the gay male hairdresser. In 1975, the hit comedy *Shampoo* featured actor Warren Beatty as a Beverly Hills hairdresser. But rather than portraying a gay hairdresser, Beatty was a "heterosexual stud . . . [a] salon cowboy who's addicted to women and wears his hair blower tucked into his jeans like a gun as he drives off on his Triumph motorbike to pay house calls, which inevitably land him in bed." In fact, the *New York Times* found that one of the "more revolutionary things in the film" was that George (Beatty's character) contradicted popular beliefs that all male hairdressers were gay, and it did so "in a quite spectacular way." Hairstyling guru Vidal Sasson even informed reporters that "Beatty has blown the whistle on us . . . [and] husbands are going to be watching us very closely." A more heterosexual image also pleased Maurice Cohen of San Francisco's St. Tropez salon who was "very happy about this movie because the first thing people think is that hairdressers are homosexual." While most stylists agreed that "George is a bit of a caricature," salon owner Peter Esser claimed "those things might happen if you looked like Warren Beatty."[28]

While the rise of unisex chain salons and "catering to people's needs" meant creating a salon that appealed to men who might have felt a bit bashful entering their mother's beauty shop, chains were also designed for working women whose tight schedules precluded high maintenance hair-dos and weekly trips to the beauty parlor. By the early 1970s, elaborately styled bouffants that were all the rage in the 1950s and 1960s fell out of fashion as "wash and wear styles" and unisex salons became popular with a younger generation of working women. Many women had indeed

grown tired of the elaborate beauty shop ritual and the time and
money spent in having their hair styled. Like San Francisco pub-
licist Ginny Kolmar, many "resented the time, and money and energy" wasted. "I went to beauty shops all my life and hated
them," complained Kolmar.[29] Indeed, the rejection of the elaborate
beauty ritual fit neatly into women's efforts to minimize certain
gender distinctions. Essayist and commentator David Bouchier
noted that "when unisex hair cutting came along, it seemed like
a great blow for sexual equality." Bouchier "had always believed
that through the ages women had been handicapped in the race
of life not (as they claimed) by male chauvinism, but by the exi-
gencies of hair care." As Bouchier put it, the unisex salon offered
women a sense of progress: "a man's haircut was a quick, low-cost
affair, over in 10 minutes. But in the bad old days women would
regularly waste whole mornings in the beauty parlor . . . and pay
a small fortune for the privilege." "The unisex salon," Bouchier
continued, "seemed the ideal solution," for it offered women the
opportunity to "receive fast haircuts and be back competing in
the corporate struggle on an equal basis with men."[30] Of course,
many such businesses were still "glitzy full service salons,"
which offered everything from permanents to pedicures. But for
working- and middle-class women managing jobs and families,
the "no frills" chain salons, which had a set number of services,
met everyone's styling needs on a limited budget and in a reasonable amount of time.[31]

The chain salon did of course have the potential to attract men
and women from various backgrounds. Like the malls in which
chains were increasingly located, however, they did not simply
blur class or race distinctions. The chain salon's more public location and emphasis on inexpensive generic cuts and styles implied
less exclusivity, less privacy, and ultimately less class. Like public transport and public schools, the chain salon's more public nature relegated it to an inferior position in an industry that remained stratified along lines of class yet ultimately defined along
lines of race. In other words, chains did not capture the essence
of the community as did the small neighborhood shop. Nor did
hairstylists readily find themselves involved in the personal lives
of their customers and communities. Hairstylists themselves expressed a similar theme in their critiques of the low-cost chain

salons, businesses they increasingly associated with cheap labor, rude customers, and exploitative management policies.[32]

At the same time, the chain salon challenged the work culture to which many stylists had grown accustomed. More specifically, the chain salon threatened to de-skill hairstylists and devalue the beauty shop as an important social institution by placing more emphasis on rapid customer turnover and less on skill, comfort, and conversation, which had long been crucial to the beauty shop ritual and worker resistance. Frances Smith, who has worked in the industry since the early 1960s, described working in a chain salon as "very stressful." Haircuts at many chains, she discovered, are timed and must not take more than fifteen minutes, while a perm, regardless of the length of hair, should take no more than two hours. And "if you don't make the quota," Smith explained, "you're out."[33] Such policies create a tremendous amount of stress on stylists. Hairstylist Janet Thompson, a white woman working in North Kansas City, found that her blood pressure began to rise after working in a chain salon. She first fixed hair in the 1950s and even though she never owned her own salon, she always enjoyed working with clients. By the 1980s, she had been out of the business for a while and began working in a chain. Rather than set appointments, Thompson recalled, customers "would sit up on this bench and wait and tap their foot," and every time she would glance over at the line of waiting customers she became especially "nervous" and "upset."[34] Leslie Peterson, a young white female stylist who has supplemented her income by cutting hair at the local prison, has found that the prisoners are often "more polite" than the average chain-store customer. At the prison, "they're so grateful. . . . They tip me with Jolly Ranchers [and other] pieces of candy." Of course, it was not just customers' disgruntled looks and actions that disturbed some stylists, but, according to Thompson, the manager who was always "rushing" the stylists and interfering with their work. Her manager had no training in styling hair, yet would "actually start getting in there" and "rinse your perms" or "help you take it down" by removing the curling rods.[35]

But it was more than just the pace of work that troubled Janet Thompson; she often found herself working longer days and not receiving adequate pay. Thompson, for example, had little control over how many clients she had each day, and several times a week she worked until ten or eleven at night. At times, she worked well over forty hours a week, but it was difficult to prove because management gave "breaks," which did not count as paid labor. "Every time that you stop and pause they don't count that on the clock . . . or if it's slow that day you can't leave [the salon]." Instead, "you've got to sit around and wait for someone to come in and that's why you can't complain about how many hours you put in." Management could simply argue "you didn't do anything for that many hours." "Until I went out on my own," confessed Thompson, "I didn't realize how much they made off of me." Leslie Peterson agreed that "the reason why the chain . . . makes it so well, is because they rip off the hairstylists who works there."[36]

Management positions have been equally problematic at chain salons. Monica Rogers complained that working at a department-store salon was "very stressful," especially during the two years she served as a productivity supervisor. "If you don't make productivity, you get called into the office which was my job." Being both a supervisor and a hairstylist was difficult, complained Rogers, because "I'm on both sides of the fence, you know, and it's kind of hard to ask the hairstylist why she's not making productivity when you know there are no customers to make productivity with." As she quickly discovered, the department store she worked at had an unusually high productivity requirement but did little to help their employees make their quota. Not only did they hire too many stylists, but they never advertised, and the salon she worked in was virtually hidden from the customers "upstairs, behind children's wear in a corner." Rogers' experiences in management were so unnerving that she would never consider managing another salon even if she had the opportunity to own the business.[37]

The high turnover rate suggests another major problem with chain salons. "Stylists are not loyal to a chain," insisted Leslie Peterson. Instead, "they go where they get the most money." This is quite different from the small salon Frances Smith owned, which she found "could run itself." "I could go out at one o'clock in the afternoon," recalled Smith, because her "newest" employee had worked for her seven years, while the other women had been there at least fifteen years. As Smith put it, "the problem with chain salons is [that] it's not you as a hairdresser. It's them as the big guy." Her daughter, Tammy, asserted that she would never work in a chain because it is just a way for the corporation to "make fast money." "You're not really creating anything," remarked Tammy. Instead "its get'm in-get'm out."[38] Because chains offer only a few services, Francis continued, "many of the girls that are working, say in the mall, all they know how to do is blow dry and cut hair. . . . If they had to put in pin curls in the hair they couldn't make it." Hairstylist Jamie Anderson, a white midwestern woman who has owned her own shop since the 1960s, insisted that she "wouldn't have that kind of salon. . . . They're impersonal and they run you through like an auction," a sharp contrast with beauty shops from earlier decades. Anderson remembered how many of her clients "would come early [just] so they could all talk. . . . A visit to the beauty salon was their time away from their children and their husbands and you know, the stress they were under."[39]

Even one of the hairstyling industry's leading publications admitted that there is a reason chain salons often conjure up the image of a "factory offering minimum services at minimal prices performed by overworked, underpaid junior stylists." *Salon News* characterized some as "'chop shops' [that] . . . lure unwitting cosmetology grads into sweat shop labor." "I've seen too many young people land in these places straight out of school. They get used—doing 10 or more heads a day—until they're burned up. Then they leave the profession for good," argued Terry Harrison, owner of a St. Louis hairstyling salon.[40] Leslie Peterson never forgot the first day she worked in a chain salon. "I did twenty-four haircuts in six hours" and thought "if this continues much longer I'm going to be insane." Janet Thompson concluded that chains purposely try to discourage workers. They try to "make you think that you aren't going to make it out there and that you're going to be back here [working in a chain.]" Thompson also argued that it is "unusual for chains to hire someone who is in their forties": "they have to have kids—younger people so that they can bend them, you know, so that they can work them for little or nothing."[41]

In order to "bend" workers and gain control of the beauty shop floor, chains have attempted to undermine the hairstylist-client

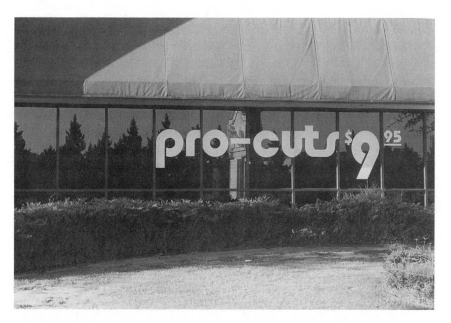

The 1990s generic chain, or what some stylists call a "chop shop." From the author's collection.

relationship, which has always been the basis of stylists' resistance. Leslie Peterson found that a chain "wants the customer going to the salon—they don't want the customer going to the stylist." Some chains, for example, demanded that stylists keep their conversations "general" and not share the intimate details of life which have traditionally been part of beauty shop culture. At times, they even required their employees to use nicknames to deter clients from following a hairstylist to another location. At one chain, Janet Thompson confronted a manager who demanded stylists "use different names . . . like Heidi or Bubbles . . . because they don't want you taking those people when you move from there." If, for example, a hairstylist told clients her real name, and "if they heard her, they would fire her," because chain stores believe all clients are their customers and "you do not take their customers."[42]

Despite an attempt to undermine customer loyalty, stylists have still managed to develop a steady clientele that offers them the opportunity to escape the rigors of chain salons. Through their skills at handling people and styling hair, Janet Thompson and a couple of her co-workers established a steady clientele, which in turn allowed them to relocate. When "I knew I was going to be quitting soon, I started getting my phone number and everything into [the customer's] hands, but they finally did catch me," although not before Thompson was able to take a substantial number of her clients elsewhere. "I didn't get them all" but "enough to go out on my own." One of Thompson's friends was even more daring. After she had officially quit working at the chain salon, "she went back that night and got the perm cards, which had all the names and numbers of customers that she had done." Now her friend owns the salon where both women are working together. It is the kind of place, Thompson was pleased to say, "where you take time with people."[43]

Of course at the same time, chain salons have continued to attract a large number of experienced stylists. Leslie Peterson had owned her own unisex salon, which was the type of salon that "offered twenty-two dollar haircuts and wine." And like many other hairstylists, she, too, had always said "oh, I'd never work for a chain. Chains are just so dirty and they screw over their employees." But when "[she] found out that [she] was pregnant," she confessed, a chain "was the first place that I came." Peterson noted that "hairstylists are known for not being able to get health insurance," but chains are "large enough to offer their employees medical and dental insurance." She was not naive, however, and knew that "basically the company is telling you that if you make some money, then I'll offer you some pennies." But for Peterson "the pennies" are what really counts. When she was on her own, Peterson admitted that she never saved money. But "with a baby on the way," she is convinced that she would always work for a chain salon. "I don't know if I would stay with [the current chain] but I will stay in some kind of chain with some type of insurance."[44]

Many stylists have also managed to carve out autonomous spaces within their new work environments. "As a stylist," Derrick Williams explained, "we sell or we don't sell. We do sloppy work or [we] don't. We're late or we leave early. I probably use thirty percent of my potential" because "I will not give [them] the satisfaction of all I've learned and that I had to pay for." Instead, he revealed that "they get what they pay for." Williams found that what he likes best about the business is that it offers him "freedom. . . . I'll have a job tomorrow, [maybe] another state, another city. I don't even have to know anybody." As a result, many veteran stylists have used chain salons to their advantage. And instead of leaving chains altogether, they negotiate and try to balance an acceptable work culture with the best wages and benefits they could possibly find by moving from one chain to another.[45]

Like the beauty shops from preceding decades, chain salons have meant long hours, demanding clients, and occupational hazards. But the work culture within the chain shops has changed in an unprecedented fashion. Regardless of whether beauty shops served a lucrative or working-class clientele, they have tended to provide personal service that includes more that just a "cut and blow dry." The chain salon's insistence on less conversation and impersonal and speedy service not only undermines the operator-client relationship, but also the comfort and intimacy that has always made the beauty ritual special and provided the basis for worker resistance. In the process, women who work in chains are less likely to speak of the artistic side of their occupation and certainly not the glamour. Instead, boredom and exhaustion have come to define the hairststylist's experience, placing her in a precarious position in an industry that relegates its least experienced and most vulnerable practitioners to positions that rival such occupations as fast food service. Like the basic burger, the generic haircut requires minimal skills and offers minimal guarantees. Unlike women from decades past, a new generation of stylists are now less likely to have acquired the different skills that make them into an "all-around" operator, further undermining their satisfaction and opportunities to influence the conditions in which they work.

Chain salons, of course, are not the only obstacle challenging women's work culture. Increasingly, women find that they are more likely to work alongside male hairstylists whose presence has long reminded female hairdressers that their status as a professional was tenuous at best. Women felt the pressure of male competition by the end of World War II, when many were being denied admittance to beauty schools because of the high numbers of returning veterans. The GI Bill of Rights, formally known as the Servicemen's Readjustment Act, gave World War II veterans an unprecedented amount of financial support, sending thousands of men to college while providing loans and allowances for subsistence, tuition, and books. Thirty-seven thousand men used the GI Bill to enter the field of beauty culture. By 1955, the percentage of men with a beauty operator's license still ranged from a meager 2 percent in large midwestern cities to an equally insignificant 3 percent on the East Coast. Yet despite the small number of men working in beauty services, they generally occupied management positions or "highly specialized occupations." By 1962, the percentage of men in the profession had climbed to 12 percent, and while they continued to dominate positions in the most exclusive salons, they were also increasingly working in the growing number of moderately priced businesses as well as chains, and again they usually occupied management/stylist positions in the cheaper salons.[46]

By the 1970s, the figure for men remained at around 10 percent, but amidst the postindustrial decline and the collapse of manufacturing jobs, working-class men often described hairdressing as one of the few occupations left that still offered lucrative wages and promotions. David Schroder argues that it was quite common in Chicago for a man to have a well-established career in hairdressing by the time he reached his early twenties, earlier than in other occupations. Of course, some men never considered hairdressing a real option, because as one hairdresser explained, it was "too faggoty." Yet many working-class men, regardless of their sexual identity, understood hairdressing as their best option. "Hell, why not enter hairdressing school?" declared one male stylist. "The only other thing I could have done was go to welding school or auto mechanics school. And I didn't like either one of those." With hairdressing, he insisted, "I had a good chance to raise myself, make some bread, get a nice apartment, and some good sounds. What the hell did I want to fuck around under a car for? It's dirty work, and besides, you can't get nowhere."[47]

Yet while hairdressing has offered men a solid career opportunity, female hairstylists are at best ambivalent about the presence of the male hairdresser. Janet Thompson, for example, captured the uncertainty frequently expressed. If she had to work with a man, she believed that hairdressing was perhaps the best occupation because most men, she argued, tended to be gay or behave in a fashion conducive to a female-dominated work environment. In contrast, a "man-man," tended to be disruptive because they were "either flirting with your customers or with you." Yet with a gay hairdresser, Thompson explained, you could still get him to do all the "manly things" like "fix electrical problems and change light bulbs," chores she and her female coworkers found a nuisance.[48]

Most female stylists, however, felt that men had an unfair advantage when it came to clients. "It's amazing what men can get by with," complained Thompson. "I've seen customers wait a long time for a male hairdresser, even if he's late . . . [the client says] 'Oh that's no problem.'" Perhaps if they are in a hurry, Thompson thought, then they will "let one of the girls cut their hair, but they will go back to [him]," whether or not he offered an excuse. Tammy Smith claimed that potential customers would even call the salon just to ask if "a man . . . works there." Leslie Peterson agreed that "men have it the easiest." "Gay men, straight men, any man has it easier . . . [and] they make better money and they make better tips." It did not matter if that man is "black, white, Asian or green . . . [because] . . . a woman thinks a man knows what a man likes to see." Peterson learned early in her career that men often carried more respect and authority than women in the minds of many clients. "Even in school they tell you if there is a guy in your shop and you have [a problem customer] who thinks the curls are too tight, or . . . the color is too red, or too blonde . . . have a man come over and say 'oh, it looks good' and they'll believe it." Most of the famous hairdressers have been men, she insisted. "Women [may] cook" Peterson declared, "but all the great chefs are men [and] that's the way it is in hairdressing."[49]

Male hairdressers have also been well aware of their personal advantage and sometimes have even boasted about how easily they could manipulate their female clients. One Chicago hairdresser revealed that one of his favorite tricks of the trade is to "test a client's hair to see if it is dry by kissing it. Women love it because they think I am kissing their hair," and lips, he continued to explain, "are the most sensitive part of your body." As he put it, "there's only one part of the body more sensitive.'" Another Chicago hairdresser believed that his female clients viewed him as "some kind of authority," which allowed him to "persuade fifty percent of his clients to do most anything—even something so important as how to vote in an election." "I frequently read or hear something, and promote it among my customers all day." He bragged that on a regular basis, he "influences [clients] on things like what kind of clothes they should wear, how they should decorate their houses, how they should landscape their yards, or what kind of kitchen cabinets they should have installed." At times, he has even instructed "his clients in such intimate matters as how to have sex with their husbands while keeping their hair in place."[50]

At the same time, female stylists argued that male hairdressers did not simply manipulate their female clients; they overindulged and pampered them. "They bend over backwards for them," complained Janet Thompson, "and even offer them coffee." Wealthier clients who are especially lonely, explained Jamie Anderson, want a man to act as if he were "personally her slave" while showering them with endless compliments and telling her "Oh, how lovely, just lovely [and] oh, you are so cute." If a man says "Oh honey, you are so beautiful," complained Leslie Peterson, "you know that a woman is throwing money at his feet." Not all men, of course, were willing to go to that much trouble to please their clients. African-American hairstylist Derrick Williams, who has served the needs of both black and white customers, asserted that he would rather work in a chain than an exclusive salon that caters to wealthy clients, because the latter involves "just too much servitude and it ain't worth it to me."[51] Williams and some female hairstylists' refusal to overindulge their clientele reflects a long history of service work and the degree to which that work has been defined in terms of gender, race, and class. Euro-American men, for example, who have generally worked in more exclusive shops and served wealthier white women are more readily defined in terms of their professional expertise and thus do not jeopardize their own position even as they pampered their clientele.

The manner in which female hairstylists described their male counterparts also suggests that the rough working-class masculinity associated with Joshua Freeman's construction workers or David Montgomery's machinists would not translate well into the beauty salon where men are expected to charm society ladies. But this should not mean that male hairdressers do not assert a "manly bearing" towards anyone who attempts to undermine their control of the beauty shop floor. Robin D. G. Kelley finds that resistance must be understood in terms of "generational" and "cultural specificity." McDonald's employees, for example, used a "spatula like a walking stick or a microphone," turned tossing trash into an "opportunity to try out . . . Dr. J moves," and with their bodies, gestures, and jokes created a more enjoyable work experience. Similarly, male hairdressers transformed "work into performance" and altered the labor process to create a more acceptable environment and experience that also reasserted male authority. But instead of the aggressive "manly bearing" upon which men relied to intimidate unruly bosses and co-workers, male hairdressers rely more heavily on their expertise, knowledge and sex appeal to assert their own version of the manly bearing.[52] Male hairdressers described themselves as artists and experts, while their clients' hair styles were nothing less than creations. In stark opposition to the image of the artist stood women whom male stylists described as "pin curler" hairdressers who do simple "bread and butter dos" and cater not to fashion but to "little, old, blue-haired ladies."[53] The owner of a Chicago beauty school understood the difference between his work and that of the kitchen beautician in terms of gender and class:

I take the customers who interest me, and the others I send to Suzie down the street. Let her do the tootsie rolls and railroad tracks. Ten years from now they will still be going to Suzie, and they will have a wonderful relationship discussing what happened in their beds the night before. Me, I am not interested in it. . . . Women seem to need gossip for mental stimulation. They chatter away and their clients approve of their work—that is what they think. But that sort of thing runs against every fiber in my body.[54]

Afros, Cornrows, and Jesus Hair

Barry Fletcher, an African-American cosmetologist and owner of the Hair Gallery in Capital Heights, Maryland, complained that the "image of the 'dumb beauty operator' is still out there." And because of its persistence, he refuses to be identified as a hairdresser, but instead considers himself a "cosmetology entrepreneur."[55]

Since the 1970s, then, changes in the industry have brought contested notions of professionalism into sharper relief by reinforcing gender and class distinctions that long defined men as professionals and women as service workers. Professional work is prestigious to a large degree even today because it is an occupation filled with members of a dominant class and culture. Thus professional status is still reserved for the most privileged, and because of women's "second sex" status, they are denied similar recognition.[56] In the hairstyling industry, men, regardless of race, occupy a disproportionate number of the jobs in exclusive salons, which enhances their position as leaders in the field of fashion. In particular, because men dominate in the more exclusive salons, the rise of chain salons, which emphasize rapid customer turnover and less conversation, have reinforced the position of men in the industry at women's expense. At the same time, the growth of chain salons has resulted in the decline of many small neighborhood shops and strained the community-based relationships upon which female hairdressers have traditionally based their status as hairdresser, confidant, and community leader. By insisting on rapid customer turnover and less conversation, chain salons directly challenge women's ability to become "more than just a hairdresser" to their clients. Instead, chains vitiate the relationship between customers and hairstylists and rigidly divide women's work from community, threatening their livelihood and identity.

The experiences of Frances Smith and her daughter Tammy offer a poignant example of a single generation of change in the hairstyling industry. In the 1960s, Francis viewed hairdressing as a glamorous occupation, a chance to escape a small Missouri farming community and enjoy what she described as the "finer things in life." Within a year, she had graduated from beauty school and worked her way into one of the most exclusive salons in the mid-Missouri area. Francis' skills at dressing hair not only helped support her husband but also provided the "main pay check" for her growing family. Her experiences at the first salon allowed her and all seven of her co-workers to open their own beauty parlors and become successful entrepreneurs. Thirty years later, her daughter Tammy quickly grew disillusioned with the occupation. While she is the only one she knows from school who still "does hair," she, too, plans to change careers in the not-so-distant future. Tammy's generation is more likely to work in a chain that offers little advancement, but even the small independent shop where Tammy works offers no more opportunity. Indeed, as her mother pointed out, "she is barely making it," and she does not find the occupation at all glamorous. Tammy does not see clients on a weekly basis, and, unlike her mother's clients who quickly became "like family," her clients tend to be "middle-class men" and "college kids" who leave in a few years. As well, Tammy "doesn't gossip much" and rejects the seemingly archaic image of the "kitchen beautician," who is often portrayed in popular films as "some poor person, smacking their jaws, and very unprofessional." Tammy and other young female stylists are caught between contesting notions of professionalism, neither of which they can easily achieve. One definition depicts men as professionals. The other is fashioned through the rituals of a women's culture, yet seems to have little place in today's unisex salons.[57]

Just as corporate America took notice of white men's hair styles and attempted to create a salon that blurred gender distinctions, manufactures and salons owners became equally interested in African-American hair styles and the profit potential. While afros and cornrows captured the attention of the nation, Afro-Sheen and the black hair-care industry attracted the attention of white corporate America. But unlike the carefree trends in Euro-American fashion that neatly fit the format of the chain salon, black hair styles remained elusive to whites. To a large degree, the problem industry leaders had in controlling the "ethnic market" reflects the ways in which notions of race and identity remain inextricably bound to hair, style, and fashion, ideas that challenge the ways in which white stylists defined their own professional identity. But the difficulty in "courting the ethnic market" also speaks to resistance. While black hair became an important means of political rebellion throughout white America, it became a highly contested terrain in the hairstyling industry. Every attempt of white businesses to attract the "ethnic market" was met with fierce resistance from the hairstylists working for them who viewed efforts to break down ethnic and racial barriers as another threat to beauty shop culture and their professional identity.

"In the 1960s and 70s, the afro was more than hair," revealed novelist Bebe Moore Campbell. "It was the symbol of black pride, a silent affirmation of African roots and the beauty of Blackness. Neither Black men nor Black women made the transition to the afro casually," she continued, "but for Black women more mental undoing was involved." For generations, young girls had stood "in front of a kitchen stove and breathed in air redolent with Dixie Peach and frying hair" as they tried to control what she had been taught was an "offending texture" that ultimately had to be "burned into submission." Campbell believed that the old standards of beauty "were a tiny, suffocating box filled with self-hatred . . . [but] The lid came off in the '60s," which became a "Time to change the definitions of nappy and kinky to mean good. Real good." But she recalled "it took more than a phone call to the hairdresser asking for Shirley Temple curls, the flip, a new look; adopting the Afro, at least initially, required making an appointment with oneself."[58]

In the late 1960s, political activist Assata Shakur also made an appointment with herself. As a young girl, Assata's grandmother taught her that "good hair was better than bad hair, meaning that straight hair was better than nappy hair," and "everybody knew you had to be crazy to walk the streets with nappy hair sticking out." But when Assata entered Manhattan Community College, she was exposed to a wealth of students from diverse backgrounds and felt she was changing along with "her concept of beauty." While she believed that a "revolutionary-thinking person" can have "hair fried up" and that someone with an afro could easily be "a traitor to Black people," she also felt that "When you wear your hair a certain way . . . you are making a statement about yourself." And for her, wearing a natural captured the essence of the Black Power Movement. The afro, Assata insisted,

was important not just because of how good it made me feel but because of the world in which i lived. In a country that is trying to completely negate the image of Black people, that constantly tells us we are nothing, our culture is nothing, i felt and still feel that we have got to constantly make positive statements about ourselves.

For African Americans, she continued, "our desire to be free has got to manifest itself in everything we do. . . . Maybe in another time, when everyone is equal and free, it won't matter how anybody wears their hair or dresses or looks."[59]

The popularity of the afro and other African-American hair styles was not limited to black women and men, however. Indeed, the afro could be bought and sold like any other commodity. Bebe Moore Campbell remembered when "The Afro went on sale for $29.95" and even "white women started wearing little fuzzy 'fros."[60] Nor was it long before white women started braiding their hair in cornrows, a style made "acceptable" in the movie *10* when white actress Bo Derek "portrayed the ultimate sex symbol." Richelle Braithwait, who worked as a cornrower at Casdulan Hairdressers in Harlem in 1980, expressed disbelief that "white women are paying $300 for a hairstyle on Park Avenue that any child in Harlem can do." But what angered African-American hairstylists most was not who was wearing cornrows, but who was being acknowledged for creating the style. It seemed that white hairstylists were receiving undeserved credit, making African Americans feel as though once again "black culture [had] been pillaged." Only a few white stylists seemed to realize what "cornrowing is: clearly a history, an art form, a source of pride," and "not just a style that may come and go."[61]

Even though African-American hair styles became increasingly popular throughout the late 1960s and '70s, many men and women failed to appreciate them. After a two-year study, Dr. Algie C. Brown, an Emory University dermatologist, reported to the American Medical Association that afros were responsible for hair loss in African Americans. Dr. Brown's study, based on twenty-five patients, asserted that extensive processing with "harsh chemicals, petroleum-based dressings, hot styling combs and special combs called picks" caused premature balding. Moreover, because the afro required an elaborate styling process, Brown argued that "those who wear Afros usually shampoo much less often than they should (about once a month)—which means a greater chance of scalp disease and increased dandruff." "We're not trying to say that the Afro hair style is bad," commented Dr. Brown, "but if it's worn bushy it's going to break off."[62]

Ironically while the "bush," which was "the final touch in an Afro," was in Brown's words an "unnatural," "unhealthy," and a "complex hairdo," the celebrated style was typically referred to as a "natural" because of the simplicity of the styling process.[63] Many black hairstylists were, of course, ambivalent about afros because they required little in the way of processing and made the hairdresser almost obsolete. "With the natural," complained one hairdresser, "women can shampoo their hair, and blow it out at home." In fact, hairdressers began pushing relaxers and more processed styles to encourage women to return to the beauty parlor ritual. Despite the impact afros had on the black-owned beauty shops, African-American hairstylists were unwilling to argue that afros were somehow harmful. Instead, they were quick to contradict the medical profession's basic assumption that the afro was somehow a highly-processed hair-do. Donald Forbang, who headed Moler Barber College on Mason Street in San Francisco, explained that "straightening and teasing were not part of the afro style" at all. Instead, the afro "is probably healthier than the old processed style." "I don't know who that guy talked to," questioned Lu Vason, owner of Oakland's tonsorial parlor, Hair-O-Scope, "but he didn't have it together." Similarly, Jasper Brown, owner of San Francisco's Do-City on Divisadero Street, agreed that it was "ridiculous . . . to single out one kind of hair styling." Vason shrewdly pointed out that the medical professional seemed less concerned about scalp problems than about the assertion of black style: "If that's the case," he asked, "how come all those women wearing bouffant hairdos, a few years ago aren't bald?"[64] Men and women who wore afros enthusiastically agreed. Charles Wynn, a key punch operator, was "very pleased" with his afro. "It brings out the most in black people. It's so together." In fact he believed, "all black people should wear naturals." And Mary Still, a film librarian, agreed that afros were "easy to take care of." But what she really wanted was a "bush like Angela Davis," because in her words, "the bush is the ultimate in Afro."[65]

Despite the heated debate over Brown's claim that afros were unhealthy, nowhere was the controversy surrounding style more dramatically played out than in the workplace. Whether it was hair, clothes, or shoes, corporations across the country insisted that any style that might offend customers or taint the company's professional image would not be tolerated. In the spring of 1974, for example, Greyhound Bus informed its drivers that "uniform and company standards must be observed." Drivers faced not only a "crack down on trouser leg width[s]," but they were also "required to undergo heel height measurements." "Heels higher than three quarters of an inch," Greyhound argued, jeopardized safety and interfered with the use of the break and gas pedals. Most troublesome, however, were afros, which the company described as an "extreme hairstyle," which disgraced the company's image and were subsequently prohibited. According to a company spokesman, "afro hairstyles . . . interfere with the proper wearing of a Greyhound cap with insignia and identification number." Because of what drivers called "nick picking regulations," the company banned dozens of Greyhound drivers from work. But veteran drivers continued to assert that the company's decisions were arbitrary and had "nothing to do with safety," suggesting that the afro somehow violated the company's image, an image Greyhound insisted must remain distinct from its black drivers.[66]

Much like the afro, cornrows were often challenged in the workplace. Dorothy Reed became a cause-célèbre after a San Francisco television station suspended her for wearing beaded cornrows, a style the station deemed "'inappropriate' for television." The station demanded that she restyle her hair in the "bouffant, swept back look" that she had previously worn and which they considered appropriate, a request Reed found "ridiculous" and "absurd." "It's a subjective decision, and for them to say, 'no cornrows or dreadlocks' is discrimination and denies me the right to express my heritage through hair style." Reed's case was resolved quickly thanks to numerous protests and the threat of a law suit. Within two weeks, she resumed her position on the nightly news after reaching a compromise in which the station allowed her to keep the braids if she removed the beads.[67] Over a decade later, Pamela Mitchell, an employee at the

Marriott hotel in Washington, D.C., was informed that she would lose her job as a reservationist "unless she did something with her hair." Mitchell's hair was also worn in long braids and reflected a sense of "creativity" and "superior workmanship." Yet the Marriott thought that Mitchell's hair did not present a "good business image," an image, Ralph Wiley argues, that was tainted by Pamela's "blackness" and "thick, tightly curling black hair."[68]

Reactions to black hair styles, especially to the afro, were not always as explicit, however. While black-owned beauty salons lost clients during the afro's heyday, white hairdressers were doing a brisk business straightening their Caucasian clients' hair. For white women, straightened hair seemed a reassuring symbol of whiteness during a period of dramatic political and cultural change. Indeed, straightening hair became such a rage that for the first time white-owned beauty shops began offering their clients "anti-permanents," while cosmetic manufacturers began selling cheap jars of home hair-straighteners designed especially for white consumers.[69] The obsession with which women straightened their hair was redolent of the Civil War era when white women who "'friz' their hair, 'a la d'Afrique'" were accused of threatening the color line.[70] In a similar fashion, at the height of the Black Freedom Movement, some white women tossed aside home permanents and started rolling their hair up on large rollers or orange juice cans to straighten their kinks.[71] Or if they wanted to really straighten their hair, they would resort to pressing it on an ironing board. Straight hair was such a craze, observed one school administrator in Connecticut, that "even girls with straight hair are ironing it to make it straighter."[72]

The controversy surrounding black hair styles suggests that men and women struggled for autonomous space and an alternative labor process on a "terrain [that] was often cultural, centering on identity, dignity, and fun." Not everyone who wore an afro was as explicitly political as Assata Shakur, but Robin D. G. Kelley urges against the "tendency to dichotomize people's lives [and] to assume that clear cut 'political' motivations exist separately from issues of well being, safety, pleasure, cultural expression, sexuality, freedom of mobility, and other facets of daily life." Instead, Kelley offers an example of his own experiences working at McDonald's. "I've never known anyone at our McDonald's to argue about wages," asserts Kelley. Instead, "What we fought over were more important things like what radio station to play," or "We even attempted to alter our ugly uniform by opening buttons, wearing our hats tilted to the side, rolling up our sleeves a certain way, or adding a variety of different accessories." But hair, Kelley finds, "was perhaps the most contested battle ground." Kelley recalls how managers insisted that "those of us without closely cropped cuts . . . wear hairnets, and we were simply not having it. . . . To net one's jheri curl, a lingering Afro, a freshly permed doo was outrageous." And it was "those battles," Kelley continues, that we waged "with amazing tenacity—and won most of the time."[73] The battle over afros and cornrows suggests that most contemporaries, like Kelley, did not dichotomize experience into political and nonpolitical spheres. Rather the afro, regardless of the context, was at the very least a challenge to the labor process, and, at the most, a dangerous symbol of a broader revolutionary agenda that conjured up violent images like those used to defame political activists.

Despite the controversy surrounding afros and cornrows, it did not diminish the interest of corporations in the consumer potential of African Americans. According to Robert Weems, white-owned corporations had largely ignored black consumers until the 1960s. Although white-owned companies had long been interested in straightening hair and bleaching skin, Weems explains that "During the 'Jim Crow' era, African Americans had monopolized the production of skin and hair products for blacks."[74] Through the early 1970s, black-owned beauty shops were virtually invisible from the standpoint of large white-owned corporations and commonly described as "a nickel and dime business," deemed unworthy of financial attention even though these businesses had long been a "pillar of the black business community" and respected as a profession. In the early 1970s, however, this began to change as white corporations began to take a much greater interest in the Johnson Products Company, which would become the first black-owned firm to appear on the American Stock Exchange.[75] As Weems argues, this was part of a larger trend that took off in the 1960s: at the height of the Black Freedom Movement, African Americans became, for the first time, an "overwhelmingly" urban population, one in which many individuals obtained a higher standard of living. Weems notes that at that time market research revealed a significant proportion of money being spent on personal care products.[76] Between 1971 and 1975, for example, the Johnson Products Company, the makers of Afro-Sheen, witnessed a dramatic increase in gross sales from thirteen million to thirty-nine million dollars. At the same time, white corporations conducted a series of studies that examined the frequency of salon visits and expenditures of black consumers. White executives were astonished to find that African-American women visited the beauty shop every two to four weeks and spent one and a half to twice as much on salon services than white clients. Less than a decade after the makers of Afro-Sheen "went public," "courting the ethnic market" became the rallying cry of the white-owned hairstyling industry. By the mid-1980s, white-owned corporations boasted both the ownership and control of the largest black hair-care franchises in the country.[77]

But "courting the ethnic market" did not come easy for the white hair-care industry. Because whites knew little about how African Americans took care of their hair and skin, Weems finds, they frequently relied on black consultants who shared crucial insights. This was especially important during the height of the Black Power Movement because white corporations seemed particularly "confused." In the early 1960s, white advertisers pushed themes that alluded to assimilation and seemed to complement the early goals of the Civil Rights Movement. But soon corporate advertising had to readjust itself to capture black nationalist sentiment and "'plug' into the soul scene."[78] By the 1980s, this marketing trend was a well-established procedure as white-owned chain salons tried to mask the color of their company with the use of Afrocentric facades. Selig and Latz, a white-dominated firm owned "Soul Scissors," "Soul Set," and "Soul Shop," forty-six salons in New York. Similarly, "Black Hair Is" was another white-owned franchise with international locations in both the United States and South Africa.[79] Yet journalist Lisa Jones found that even though manufacturers such as Shark Products used "afrochic" gimmicks and advertise in *Ebony* and *Essence*, they ultimately chose watermelon for the company's signature-fragrance and hence revealed the underlying racist assumptions the company held about the potential clients they were so desperately trying to attract.[80]

At the level of the salon, industry leaders were enthusiastic about the potential profit of the "ethnic market." According to Robert Mugnai, publisher of *American Salon*, there were "two major profit centers . . . developing in the Professional Salon Industry." One is the "increasingly important youth market which are clients from the ages of 17 to 24." The other is what he called "the challenging ethnic market, which includes Blacks, Hispanics, Orientals and those clients with special ethnic differences in their hair and skin types," a market potentially more profitable than white markets. To "court the ethnic market," Mugnai suggested that white salon owners open earlier and close later to meet the needs of black working women, try to provide an "inviting atmosphere" through the "presentation of familiar ethnic brand name products," and hire "cosmetologists who are familiar with Black skin tone differences, hair textures and styling requirements." White-owned salons were in fact "training and hiring stylists who can perform services for Black clients." "A decade ago, it would have been doubtful that clients could find personal care services for Whites and Blacks under one salon roof," the editorial explained. "Now it is becoming common place particularly in commercial or industrial districts." "Courting the ethnic market," the editorial claimed, had produced a "merging of cultures," but it also argued that "the one-chair salon that has been the bulwark of the ethnic salon business" was on the "wane."[81]

"Courting the ethnic market" did more than change the name of white-owned salons and advertising campaigns, however; it also imposed structural changes within the salon itself. A generation earlier, most white hairstylists never saw black clients. Frances Smith recalled that in the 1960s, "we didn't do blacks. We were prejudice I guess you would say because you had some that would try to get in." Most white women of Smith's generation did not work with or know of any African-American hairdressers. Frances, for example, was unaware of the locations of black-owned beauty parlors in her own town but suspected they were in someone's "back room."[82] And in large cities, if an African-American woman entered a department store salon, she was ushered to the back of the salon where she met a "little black lady in

184 the back, in the corner, in the dark, locked up with her stove and

the back, in the corner, in the dark, locked up with her stove and comb, not exposed at all . . . because . . . they used to say the hair would smell and bother the white clientele."[83]

By the 1970s, white hairstyling trade journals began to feature black hair styles, and, for the first time, beauty schools were teaching a younger generation of white hairstylists techniques used to create popular black hair styles. Frances Smith's daughter Tammy, for example, worked extensively with African-American clients in her cosmetology courses even though she has only had a few black clients over the years. Chain salons have even attempted to bring black and white customers under the same roof.[84] Monica Rogers, who started working in the early 1980s in a southern-based chain, frequently did what she referred to as "black curls," and she remarked that it was primarily in chains where she worked more closely with black stylists and customers. Even within the last few years, Rogers has noticed a dramatic increase in the number of black clients. Moreover, an older generation of white hairdressers who were never trained in "black hair styles" began attracting the occasional African-American client. But black customers did not assume that older hairstylists had the expert knowledge needed to work with "black hair" and sometimes became the stylists' coaches. In the 1950s, Janet Thompson, did not learn how to work with "black hair" but instead an African-American client explained to her in meticulous detail how to "use a big rod and a strong perm" to straighten her hair.[85]

Yet despite the industry's attempt to "court the ethnic market" and the claims of major publications that white salons had successfully attracted black clients, Derrick Williams insisted that the industry remains "about as segregated as church." Hairdressing is the "most segregated business in the country," in part because many white customers simply refuse to have black stylists cut and style their hair. Even when white customers consented to a black stylist, Derrick Williams claimed that at times you could still sense their discomfort. "When you're behind the chair year after year you get vibes. . . . I don't care what their mouth says you can feel it. The body tenses. I mean the erector pili stand up."[86]

Still, Williams has established a white clientele. "Depending on what part of the country you are in," he found, "many white

clients feel quite comfortable with a black hairdresser." He attrib- 185
uted his success at attracting white customers to his skill at cutting hair and making conversation. But he also saw it as part of a
larger pattern in which white people have come to "expect" service from African-American laborers. "Ancestrally," Williams
pointed out, African Americans have always been the ones "who
did the work and who served them."[87]

White customers are not the only reason hairdressing has remained so segregated, however. Over the years, Derrick Williams
had become familiar with the way white stylists often "look at the
black customer" and had reached the conclusion that an African
American who relies on a white hairstylist is "really a fool" because white hairstylists "damn near hate to touch your head."
Frances Smith, for example, declared that she possesses neither
the skills nor the tools to work with African-American clients
whose hair she described as being "like a fishing line" or "just
like a piece of wire." "Unless they're a little mixed and have better hair," Francis preferred not to work with "black hair" and believed that African Americans "need [instead] to go to black salons." And, "oriental hair," she complained, "will ruin your scissors, because it's thick and heavy." In a similar fashion, her
daughter Tammy Smith confessed "that if there was one thing I
hated in school it was doing jheri curls." Tammy admitted that
she felt "nervous" working with African-American customers
because they use "totally different" product lines, many of
which, she explained, are lye-based and can easily harm the hair
and skin if administered incorrectly. As well, Tammy pointed out
that Africans Americans use different terminology to describe the
same process. "Like a perm to them is a straightener." And regardless of the procedure, "you have to be so careful because their
skin is so sensitive I don't even like to mess with it."[88]

Attitudes like these have convinced many African Americans to
simply avoid white stylists. "Most black people will not trust a
white hairstylist to do their hair," declared Leslie Peterson. As a
manager of a chain that hired both black and white stylists, she
had witnessed firsthand the consumer choices of black clients.
But being "half Japanese," she was also keenly aware of the racial
dynamics of the salon. "Black people don't consider me white
. . . [but] mixed," she explained. "So if I'm standing there with

someone white . . . [and] it's me or it's her . . . they are going to pick me." "I have this coarse oriental hair," what she called her "little advantage." And it is assumed "that I know a little bit more about their hair" than the white stylists.[89] Other African-American clients tried out a white stylist but ended up going back to the stylist who knew how to handle their hair. In New Haven, Connecticut, for example, Henri Sumner found that his one-operator salon successfully competes with large department store salons in a "city that devours most small businesses." Many of his customers initially went to the department store chain, but, because the store's white manager "knew nothing about Black culture hair" and insisted on using products that caused damage to the client's hair, many of his customers suffered "chemical abuse" at the department store or other "white-product oriented salons."[90] Other black women continued to see a white stylist whom "they think will do a better job," but eventually ended up going back to the black stylist from time to time to repair the damage. Derrick Williams' mother, for example, had a regular customer who would come to her shop "with her hair messed up every single time." As soon as his mother got her hair to "come in," Williams continued, "there she goes [off] . . . to the same hairdresser that her golf friends go see" who are friends "from the job and all white." This woman, Williams asserted, "wants to be like [her white golf friends and] though she never can be—she keeps trying."[91]

The skill and knowledge required to do "black hair" certainly affected the relative position of white women in the industry, unlike the generation of women who became hairdressers before the 1970s. Tammy Smith, for example, admitted that she "envies people who do black hair." "I'm not educated well enough on it, but I think it would be awesome to watch." Similarly, while working in a chain salon, Monica Rogers often did "black curls," which were popular a few years ago, but "some of these new styles that black ladies are wearing I couldn't begin to do anything like that. . . . I just sit and watch and I'm just amazed." The intricacy of the styles has also usually meant better pay. Leslie Peterson thought that "black-owned shops do better . . . because the hair sets are so intricate." "They've got to charge more money," agreed Tammy Smith, "I mean it takes six hours to do some of those procedures, and it's much harder than our perms and colors."[92]

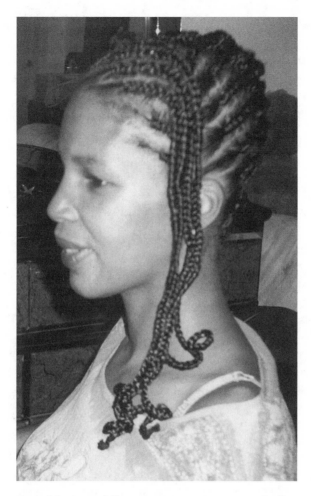

Terry Morris modeling contemporary cornrows. Styling time approximately three hours. Hair designer: Latonya Rene Sharp. Courtesy of Terry Morris.

Not all of the intricate styles favored by African Americans are stylist driven, however. "It used to be a rich person's thing [style]," noted Derrick Williams, "but now you find more and more that wealthy people are pretty plain." Instead, the "most creative work is being done in black hair." Leslie Peterson has found that most African-American customers who frequent the chain salon she manages do not want simple haircuts that are pictured on the salon's walls, but demand "the lines like Arsenio [Hall] had or . . . different, more intricate styles." Derrick Williams explained how the body often becomes "the concentration of attention [and] so attention to detail—clothes, hair, makeup [is important.]" "Hair in this country it means something. It could be a social-political barometer to measure things by." "What is underground now," he continued "will become mainstream later . . . and usually it comes from deviant lifestyles and you know impoverished neighborhoods because those people have nothing but their body so the body becomes a signpost."[93]

The intricate styles and their appropriation as a form of resistance along with the racist attitudes of many white stylists have simply meant that the "ethnic shops" industry leaders claimed were on the "wane" have continued to flourish. Indeed, many "older traditional black salons deny that there has been much of an impact on their business as a result of the white chains." Cardozo Sisters, "one of the oldest and most prosperous salons in Washington, D.C," maintains a loyal following of "socialites and sorority members" as well as Howard University students and employees. In a more modest setting in Los Angeles, Roxanne Huapaya, a hairdresser at Elana's Beauty Salon on Avenue 26, found that most of her customers live in the surrounding neighborhood and "are extremely loyal." According to Huapaya "there are a few salons in the neighborhood and we are all busy." In fact, in April 1995 *Black Enterprise* declared that "black-owned salons are gaining financial clout in the ethnic consumer market."[94] Cynthia Santiago, a hairdresser at Winston's on Melrose in Los Angeles, claimed that "There is a renaissance in black hair care" today, and "it has to do with the technology available to deal with black hair." "Black women," Huapaya continued, "have traditionally sought salons skilled in dealing with their special beauty problems." Today there are "scores of salons to choose from" that offer those services, "ranging from tiny neighborhood beauty shops on Crenshaw Boulevard to trendy West Los Angeles salons like those owned by hairdressers John Atchinson and Thaddeus Winston." Thaddeus Winston, who started out as a barber in Indiana in the 1960s, now owns his own salon on Melrose. Winston hires several stylists who are skilled in weaving and braiding, services hard to find in most chains and white-owned salons because, as Derrick

Williams points out, they violate the corporation's notion of what
it means to be a "family salon." Because hair weaving and other
beauty treatments may take several hours, Winston is also adding
private rooms with televisions in the salon and is planning to
open a beauty school specifically designed to teach stylists how
to care for black hair. Santiago calls it "salon bondage." Black
women demand intricate styles and weaves, styles "they can't do
. . . themselves so they need places like [Winston's]" and the thousands of small shops that specialize in black hair styles.[95]

The "renaissance" these stylists describe and the intricate
weaves, braids, and other processes required for African-American women's hair styles not only demand a considerable amount
of skill, but have allowed beauty shops to remain an important location for women's culture, what Patricia Hill Collins calls
"spheres of influence," one that helps women transcend daily life
and cope with "the simultaneity of [the] oppression they experience."[96] Beauty shops, for example, empower women by allowing
them the space to exchange information, goods, and services crucial to day-to-day survival. As Judith Miller found, women "go to
the beauty shops first and [then] they don't need to go anywhere
else." Her own work as a hairdresser has always involved much
more than styling her clients' hair. On a regular basis she reminds
her older patrons to visit the doctor, passes messages from one
client to the next, and listens closely for gossip detailing the
whereabouts of her clients' children. For the past two decades,
Derrick Williams' mother's shop has operated in a similar fashion
in Seattle, Washington. "When I go to my mom's shop," Williams
explained, "I find out who's died. I find out who's going to college, who's graduated from college, who got a good job, who's
in prison. You find out a lot of information is traded there:
job searching, networking happens, social events." At times,
"someone will come through from church selling dinners and
lunches or political things." The beauty shop, Williams insists,
"makes a good pedestal to shape, formulate, and exchange ideas."
"Like if Mr. Farrakhan is coming to town . . . or if something's
going on . . . we're selling tickets." The beauty shop provides "a
direct link because there are only so many institutions [in black
communities] that are alive and hold access." "You've got the
church, the hairdresser, [and there] might be a greasy spoon,"

Afros, Cornrows, and Jesus Hair

but Williams explained that "there is not a lot in those black communities."[97]

Ultimately, the central role of the beauty shop in community life and the services most shops offer have allowed hairstylists to establish more intimate and personal relationships with their clients that extend beyond the shop and into the community. "In a small salon," asserted Irma Milligan, of Fort Wayne, Indiana's Southside, "you become someone special to your patrons. My regular customers call for help much like they would call a family doctor." Milligan frequently went "into homes to fix hair for mothers who can't find baby sitters" or to style "hair for clients who are ill." On occasion she has even "gone to funeral parlors to fix hair on [her] elderly patrons who have died." "I take care of entire families and know everyone on a first-name basis." "And unlike large salons, we can 'carry' our regular customers during lean weeks." Milligan admitted that she "may not be an expert at management," but she does "know how to make people feel good," and that is "why the small salon will always be home."[98]

The demand for salons that "cater to distinct cultural and ethnic groups" has also "risen sharply" in the 1980s and 1990s among new immigrant communities. Gahin Choi, who is considered a leader in the Los Angeles Asian beauty community, founded Gahin House, a "favorite gathering place for Korean women." His salon has become part of a tradition for Korean brides, who "spend the day before their wedding being pampered at the salon." Jino Son, a hairdresser at Gahin, insisted that "there are more than 100 salons in the Korean section of Los Angeles. And, it seems that new ones are opening up every month." New immigrants not only feel "more comfortable obtaining beauty services from someone who speaks their language and understands their stylistic preferences," but these shops "are also busy because the neighborhood beauty salon has traditionally been a gathering place for women to meet and socialize."[99]

The tremendous growth in the hairstyling industry that caters to new immigrants has also meant employment opportunities for many women who have a limited amount of money to spend on a formal education. In 1988, Los Angeles County issued 56,467 cosmetology licenses, an increase of approximately 1,000 a year since the early 1980s. In 1988, Southern California reported 13,921 establishments and 114,700 licensed cosmetologists. A substantial part of that increase reflects the number of new immigrants. This is quite different from the 1950s and 1960s when most minority-owned schools were at best elaborate salons where women typically became licensed through an apprenticeship. According to Jeff Wier, a legislative analyst for the California State Board of Cosmetology, the occupation appeals to new immigrants because "there are very few entry level positions where you can get into it quickly, make a living and feed your family." In California, for example, immigrants and non-English speakers often choose cosmetology courses because they are relatively inexpensive, ranging from $2,500–$6,000, and require only a tenth-grade education or a passing grade on an equivalency test. According to the *Los Angeles Times*, "Aruni Blount's Beauty School roster reads like a meeting of the United Nations' General Assembly." Most Southland beauty colleges teach cosmetology classes in English and Spanish as well as in Thai, Vietnamese, Korean, and Japanese. Many of Los Angeles' beauty colleges have students from El Salvador, Trinidad, Nicaragua, Africa, Thailand, Malaysia, Indonesia, Hong Kong, Taiwan, Japan, Cambodia, and Vietnam, and many of the non-English speaking students bring interpreters with them when they take their state board exams.[100]

For African-American women, the beauty business also continues to offer an escape from other service industries where negotiating space and autonomy seems more difficult. Judith Miller admitted that until she became a hairdresser, she never could hold down a job. "I would change jobs like people change shoes or I should say underclothes. I think I've done just about everything. I worked in a bank, as a secretary, as a waitress, a hostess, [in] a dress shop—you name it, I've done it." But in 1986, Miller opened her own business and found out how "wonderful" it is "to find something you like to do." Similarly, Angela Roberts at the age of sixteen began working in a fast-food franchise where she spent the next fifteen years. "It seemed like an eternity," Roberts recalled, and even though she attended the McDonald's Hamburger University and had "excellent ratings," McDonald's never promoted her to the position of first manager. "The time I was there I never saw any prejudice toward me, but I believe being black and female I was not going to get a store." While

Roberts was pregnant with her third child, she and her husband decided that it would be better for her to end her tenure at McDonald's. "It might have been a bad decision," Roberts confessed, "but mentally it worked out much better," for she was able to transfer her managing skills to the beauty business and eventually establish her own business first in her home and then downtown.[101]

The increasing prevalence of African-American hairstylists should not suggest, however, that success comes easier for African Americans. "If you take a black worker in any profession," argued Derrick Williams "they've got to walk twice as fast as the other worker just to get less than the same bill." Nor does owning your own business guarantee complete autonomy. Black-owned businesses frequently are subjected to white supervision, intrusion, and harassment. "Word travels fast," when a "black person opens a business" in a small, white midwestern town, insists Angela Roberts. Roberts found that her own beauty shop quickly became the focus of town gossip until another African-American woman opened a salon down the street. Then attention shifted toward the new business whose owner, according to Roberts, was less discreet. Roberts believed that her business escaped harm because her own demeanor was rather "conservative" and did not upset the "town fathers." But another black businesswoman was immediately distrusted, Roberts recalled, primarily because she had a "flashy style" and wore "long, super blonde hair." As a result, "they began giving her a hard time and even broke her front window." After Judith Miller's business became successful, an undercover cop was sent to pose as a customer in an attempt to catch "drug dealers and pushers." While Miller readily dismissed the police investigation as any real threat to her livelihood, she found other white-controlled institutions much more problematic. Despite being a successful entrepreneur, Miller was repeatedly denied a loan. "Unlike doctors, lawyers or nurses, who were treated with respect," Miller found that banks characterized her as a "wishy-washy" hairdresser who could not be trusted. It was not until she found "a banker whose own daughter was a hairdresser, that she secured a loan for her house."[102] Securing a loan is not an isolated problem either, explained Andre Christburg, co-owner of a salon in Montgomery,

Alabama. He too, had problems securing loans and heard it was a
common problem. According to Christburg, "at some banks, it is
easier to get a 7,000 dollar loan for a car, than it is to get the same
loan for a minority business."[103]

The demise of America's manufacturing base and the prevalence of drugs has also affected the "ethnic salon." Neighborhoods in Harlem, Camden, New Jersey, Cleveland's East Side and
Boston's Roxbury, just to name a few, have suffered disproportionately because of the ongoing deinvestment and deindustrial-
ization of America's inner cities. Forty years ago Chicago's "63rd
Street was called 'Miracle Mile' by local merchants vying for
space and a piece of the pie." In the 1960s, argues Loïc Wacquant,
there were 800 businesses, including restaurants, banks, hotels,
houses, taverns, and ballrooms. Since the 1970s "lumber yards,
print shops, garages, and light manufacturing enterprises have
[all] disappeared." Instead, abandoned buildings, broken side-
walks, boarded-up storefronts, and debris fill the eighteen by
four block area. "Fewer than 90 commercial establishments remain," and Wacquant explains, most of these businesses are "tiny
eating places, beauty parlors, and barber shops, apparel, food,
and liquor outlets."[104]

In the process, argues Derrick Williams, the "advent of crack"
has devastated "urban communities in the inner-city neighborhoods," and "some of the legitimacy of the [beauty salon] to be
solid for the community has kind of shifted." "A lot of stylists,"
Williams claimed, "were getting involved in the illegal drug
business and a lot of people in the 1980s lost their business behind that mess." As a result, much of the "underclass" do not
even go to shops to get their hair done. Yet it is the "black underclass," Williams argued, "[that] really needs that information say
for AIDS [prevention]," which the beauty shop has traditionally
offered communities. Instead, Williams insisted, "if they get anything done—somebody's braiding [hair] in their kitchen."
"You've got a black guy here in Columbia[, Missouri], who is suppose to be a good haircutter and where does he cut hair? In the
park in Columbia and a lot of people know about him." So while
in a "middle-class" beauty salon where you "get school teachers,
ministers, those who work for police departments, big-county
jobs, [and] the military—you get a lot of information exchanged

there and it's valuable to the community." But in a "ghetto shop . . . all that's going on there is the exchange of money, drugs, information on stolen merchandize, and things like that. . . . I witnessed it in Los Angeles, South Central Los Angeles, San Francisco, Palo Alto, all up and down the West Coast. I've seen it in San Antonio and it's right here [in mid-Missouri]."[105]

Yet while the outlook of these "ghetto shops" is grim, they still remain crucial for survival because they continue to serve as a place to exchange "hot items." In large urban areas, Judith Miller explained that beauty shops are filled with "drugs, stolen goods, food stamps, and . . . plain people—just begging." "But the thing you have to understand," insisted Williams, "is that the black community is underground. All across America it's an underground economy." "There is hardly a black person I know who depends solely on their job for income," he continued. "I'm not saying they all sell drugs. I'm saying you learn to survive," which he thought had become "especially important in the last twenty to twenty-five years."[106]

Beauty shops also continue to play an important role in the health of women and have recently extended themselves in the fight against AIDS and other health problems. In the 1990s, for example, the University of California along with the state department of health initiated outreach programs designed to tap into the beauty shop's legacy as a community provider. Both programs are "based on the idea that African-American and Latina women feel more comfortable talking about the intimate details of their lives in hair salons than in doctor's offices." With these programs, more than a hundred hair salons are informing clients of sexual health issues and passing out AIDS information and condoms. In South Carolina, a similar program has been in operation since the late 1980s inspired by stylist and AIDS activist DiAna DiAna. As well, outreach programs through beauty shops are targeting other diseases that hit low income and African-American women the hardest. Breast cancer, for example, which kills African-American women at a rate 50 percent higher than among white women, has reached alarming rates, and, in places like San Diego, pilot programs are being established in beauty shops where stylists are given specific information regarding breast self-examinations, the necessity of mammograms, and connections between weight loss, smoking, and cancer rates. The growth of these programs reflects not only the poverty that disproportionately affects women of color but also the legacy of beauty shop culture and Jim Crow, which have limited the access women of color have had to medical practitioners and other professionals that they can afford and trust.[107]

Since the 1970s, then, there have been several dramatic changes in the industry that have not only profoundly shaped the labor process but also the ways in which hairstylists understand their own professional identity. As Derrick Williams notes, "this business is not the business it used to be." Williams's sense of change reflects not only concerns over the rise of chain salons, which have de-skilled and depersonalized the beauty shop ritual, but specifically corporate America's attempt to "court the ethnic market."[108] "White people have borrowed many things from black people over the years," Ralph Wiley insists, "but black people never thought they'd be coming for our hair."[109] Ironically, corporate attempts to homogenize the industry and blur race and ethnic boundaries have brought these distinctions into sharper focus. To a large degree, this reflects the nature of the industry. Unlike the production of fast food where the labor process is distinct from the product served, a hair style can not be separated from the hands that create it. In other words, because notions of race, class, and gender have so profoundly shaped the work culture of the salon, it was not simply a matter of attracting black customers. Corporate America also had to meet black and white stylists' needs and expectations. For nearly a century, the white hairdressing industry, from the level of the national association to the neighborhood shop, fashioned its own politics of exclusion and preserved a culture of whiteness by ignoring African-American contributions. This assured white female stylists that although they may never be considered professionals in the eyes of men, they would never be relegated to the back of the department store's salon with the black stylists. But since the 1970s, African American hairstylists have assumed a much more prominent position in the industry and not simply as "shampoo girls," but as highly skilled artisans. Unlike their predecessors, then, white stylists today are less likely to have the luxury of a "politics of exclusion" upon which to base their professional identity.

Yet it has been more than racism and white obstinacy that has allowed African-American women to successfully manipulate this rapidly changing industry. African-American salons continue to thrive because they play a vital role within black communities and because of the intricate styles black women continue to wear. To be sure, white women have also retained important links to their communities, but for African-American businesses, especially beauty salons, "the community has always been like a Rock of Gibraltar"[110] Despite recent changes in the industry, women refuse to relinquish their relationships with their clients or their community as they fashion their own understanding of professionalism and an identity that reflects rather than undermines a women's culture and embraces rather than rejects the racial and ethnic character of the community. The small neighborhood shop offers women a special kind of prestige that is community-based and can not be easily imposed, replicated, or even undermined. And it is within these small shops that a women's culture not only survives, but often provides the makings of an oppositional culture that in turn allows hairstylists to make their own kind of waves.

Conclusion

O n her birthday in 1994, Elizabeth Hewlett "wanted nothing fancier than a shampoo, blow-dry and possibly a haircut." But Bloomingdale's fashionable salon rejected her "simple request." Reportedly the white hairstylist refused to serve Hewlett because of her "black hair." "They would not even answer her question about whether she could have it cut and washed at the same time," stated Maryland lawyer, Stan Derwin Brown. In August 1996, after settlement talks failed to resolve the situation, Hewlett filed a class-action suit against Bloomingdale's apparent pattern of racial discrimination.[1]

Elizabeth Hewlett's experience offers a poignant example of many of the issues facing beauty salons today and throughout hairdressing's history in the twentieth century. When Hewlett was denied a simple shampoo and the "possibility of a haircut," the Bloomingdale's hairstylist refused not only to accept her business, but also the potential relationship that accompanied a visit to the beauty shop. Bloomingdale's hairstylist's unwillingness to work with "black hair" ultimately meant that the stylist was resisting the social interactions that had come to characterize the labor process. Even the relatively brief moments spent washing and cutting a customer's hair require a certain degree of intimacy. At the very least, the hairstylist is expected to make conversation, feign some interest in the client's well-being, or perhaps even lend a sympathetic ear to her personal problems.

Throughout the twentieth century, the intimacy associated with the client-hairdresser relationship has served as the cornerstone of a thriving women's culture. In their beauty shops, operators and clients shared stories and advice about families, jobs, and relationships, and beauticians even performed special favors for their clients outside of their shops and after hours. As a result, trips to the beauty shop created bonds that helped women cope with the different problems they confronted throughout the life cycle and produced an intimacy that has allowed beauty shops to create an oppositional culture that reflected the everyday politics of women's lives as well as larger community concerns. During the Depression, for example, the beauty shop provided philanthropic aid to help customers and their families deal with the hard times they faced. In working-class communities, beauty shops have often provided a place to exchange goods and services or establish networks that might lead to job contacts. Beauty shops, then, provided the location for a women's culture that could in turn create a culture of resistance. For African-American women this oppositional culture offered them some of the resources necessary to take on America's system of apartheid. Throughout the twentieth century, the beauty shop was one of the few black-owned businesses able to successfully defy white capital and white control. Thus, beauty shops afforded a unique opportunity to work and socialize within an exclusively black-owned institution. Such an environment provided a climate of trust and security and a safe space to exchange information, formulate ideas, and challenge larger structures of oppression.

At the same time, the intimacy of the operator-client relationship allowed hairdressers to more readily confront challenges to their own work culture and even establish their own businesses. Developing a loyal clientele provided the greatest sense of job security and even a stronger sense of satisfaction. A hairstylist with steady clients could more easily resist arbitrary management decisions and demand better wages and working conditions; and if need be, she could even refuse to accept clients she found objectionable. If a hairdresser found her working conditions too unbearable, the intimate relationships she had established with her clients allowed her to take them to a competing salon down the street or maybe to her own newly established business. In the process, the intimacy derived from such relationships and the hairstylist's involvement in larger community affairs allowed her to assert an identity and a sense of professionalism that revolved around the community and the sociability of the beauty salon.

Yet while the intimacy that characterized the beauty shop transformed it into an important community and social institution, it also produced a number of rigid boundaries that made it easier for that intimacy to flourish. Throughout most of the twentieth century and in most beauty shops, one such boundary revolved around gender. Although the beauty shop initially developed over a struggle for homosocial space, and there have always been some beauty shops and barber shops with both a steady male and female clientele, the beauty business was a predominantly sex-segregated industry. In fact, it was not until the 1970s and the rise of unisex chain salons that men assumed a more conspicuous role in the beauty salon as hairdressers and as clients. Men's growing presence did, at times, compromise the day-to-day ways in which women had grown accustomed to running their shops. But many other women were pleased with the addition of a male presence and embraced the intimacy that many male hairstylists had to offer. Male hairdressers have even boasted about the use of titillation to cultivate a large female following and the sensual manner in which they handled their female clients.

Of course while industry leaders and shop owners were able to successfully negotiate the issue of gender, racial boundaries proved more resistant. Much of the ambivalence white hairstylists expressed reflected the ways in which they constructed their understanding of "black hair." Stylists often complained that they were unfamiliar with black hair-care products and techniques and that "black hair" was too coarse and unmanageable. Yet the history of the hairdressing industry suggests that their complaints reflected more than an unfamiliarity with "black hair." Their ambivalence grew out of a broader legacy of exclusion and an age-old taboo about the intermingling of the races. Like gender, race was a defining characteristic of the modern beauty shop. As women began to search out their own beauty space, they inevitably found their way into barber shops—some of which were black-owned and operated. Some states enacted Jim Crow laws to ensure the separation of black men and white women. In other states, the beauty shop simply evolved out of a larger pattern of racial segregation and the violence that generally

Conclusion

accompanied it. Either way, white stylists and clients embraced and helped create a racially exclusive beauty shop that played an important role in the development of a larger culture of whiteness around which men and women fashioned their identity. By the late 1960s and early 1970s, shop owners and industry leaders became more interested in the black hair-care industry's profit potential. But they have never been able to fully undermine the intimacy that has structured the relationships between hairdresser and client, relationships that profoundly shaped beauty shop culture. The actions and attitudes of Bloomingdale's stylists reflect the degree to which the labor process is bound to this intimacy and a clear articulation of the kind of racial segregation that will always affect the hairdressing industry at its most intimate level as long as racism continues to shape American culture and society.

Ironically, while chain salons' advertising campaigns have tried to mask distinctions of race, corporate America's growing influence has only reinforced race and class hierarchies. Although exclusive salons like Bloomingdale's continue to flourish, most chains are at the other end of the scale and are associated with shopping malls and other service jobs. The bonds of intimacy that have shaped the history of hairdressing have offered a measure of resistance against corporate efforts to further de-skill service workers, lower their wages, and undermine their control, yet many hairstylists increasingly face conditions that rival that of fast-food work. Indeed, high turn-over rates and occupational burnout have come to characterize much of the industry. At the same time and most important of all, the latest threats to beauty workers and their shop cultures have much broader implications that stretch beyond the workplace. As a century of hairdressing has shown, the beauty shop, the worker, and the customer have been at the forefront of community change and institution building. While some of these institutions have been based on exclusion and upheld the status quo, others have provided rare resources and have been geared toward social change. Thus corporate trends in hairdressing have much broader implications that remind us that attempts to undermine worker control affect larger social and community efforts designed to protect individual freedom and civil rights.

Conclusion

Notes

Notes to the Introduction

1. For a discussion of "porch culture" see Jacquelyn Dowd Hall, *Like A Family: The Making of a Southern Cotton Mill World* (Chapel Hill: University of North Carolina Press, 1987), 170–71.

2. On male culture see, for example, Roy Rosenzweig, *Eight Hours for What We Will: Workers and Leisure in an Industrial City, 1870–1920* (Cambridge: Cambridge University Press, 1983). On fraternal orders see Mary Ann Clawson, *Constructing Brotherhood: Class, Gender, and Fraternalism* (New Jersey: Princeton University Press, 1989); Mark Carnes, *Secret Ritual and Manhood in Victorian America* (New Haven: Yale University Press, 1989). On urban amusements and same-sex relationships see George Chauncey, *Gay New York: Gender, Urban Culture, and the Making of the Gay Male World, 1890–1940* (New York: Basic Books, 1994). On the rise of commercial institutions and working-class women's leisure see Kathy Peiss, *Cheap Amusements: Working Women and Leisure in Turn-of-the-Century New York* (Philadelphia: Temple University Press, 1986).

3. On the struggle over public space see Randy D. McBee, *Dance Hall Days: Intimacy and Leisure among Working-Class Immigrants in the United States* (New York: New York University Press, forthcoming).

4. Marjorie Stewart Joyner, interview by Michael Flug, Vivian G. Harsh Research Collection of Afro-American History and Literature, The Carter G. Woodson Regional Library, Chicago, Il.

5. Lois W. Banner, *American Beauty* (Chicago: University of Chicago Press, 1983), 13–14. For a discussion of the ways in which race defines notions of beauty see Kathy Peiss, "Making Faces: The Cosmetics Industry and the Cultural Construction of Gender, 1890–1930," *Genders* 7 (spring 1990); Kathy Peiss, *Hope in a Jar: The Making of America's Beauty Culture* (New York: Metropolitan Books, 1998); Noliwe M. Rooks, *Hair Raising: Beauty, Culture, and African American Women* (New Brunswick: Rutgers University Press, 1996).

6. Barbara Melosh, *"The Physician's Hand": Work Culture and Conflict in American Nursing* (Philadelphia: Temple University Press, 1982), 20.

7. See, for example, Robert Weems, *Desegregating the Dollar: African American Consumerism in the Twentieth Century* (New York: New York University Press, 1998).

8. Susan Porter Benson, *Counter Cultures: Saleswomen, Managers, and Customers in American Department Stores, 1890–1940* (Urbana: University of Illinois Press, 1986); Dorothy Sue Cobble, *Dishing It Out: Waitresses and Their Unions in the Twentieth Century* (Urbana: University of Illinois Press, 1991); Greta Foff Paules, *Dishing It Out: Power and Resistance among Waitresses in a New Jersey Restaurant* (Philadelphia: Temple University Press, 1991); Wendy Gamber, *The Female Economy: The Millinery and Dressmaking Trades, 1860–1930* (Urbana: University of Illinois Press, 1997).

Notes to Chapter 1

1. Gladys L. Porter, *Three Negro Pioneers in Beauty Culture* (New York: Vantage Press, 1966), 15–18.

2. Kobena Mercer, "Black Hair/Black Style," in *Out There: Marginalization and Contemporary Cultures*, ed. Russell Ferguson et al. (Cambridge: Massachusetts Institute for Technology, 1990), 248.

3. For examples of African-American beauty parlors in the antebellum period see Rooks, *Hair Raising*, 24; for African hairstyling traditions see A'Lelia Perry Bundles, *Madam C. J. Walker* (New York: Chelsea House, 1991), 65–66.

4. Esi Sagay, *African Hairstyles: Styles of Yesterday and Today* (London: Heinemann, 1983), 1, 11, 106.

Notes to the Introduction

5. Rooks, *Hair Raising*, 25. Amol Lincoln originally quoted in Elizabeth Fox-Genovese, *Within the Plantation Household: Black and White Women of the Old South* (Chapel Hill: University of North Carolina Press, 1988), 216. Former slave descriptions of turbans quoted in Shane White and Graham White, *Stylin': African American Expressive Culture from Its Beginnings to the Zoot Suit* (Ithaca: Cornell University Press, 1998), 61. On the history of slave women see Deborah Gray White, *Ar'n't I A Woman: Female Slaves in the Plantation South* (New York: Norton, 1985).

6. Orlando Patterson, *Slavery and Social Death: A Comparative Study* (Cambridge: Harvard University Press, 1982), 61–62. On slavery see also George Rawick, *From Sundown to Sunup: The Making of the Black Community* (Westport, Conn.: Greenwood Press, 1972).

7. Patterson, *Slavery and Social Death*, 61–62.

8. White and White, *Stylin'*, 55–56.

9. Harriet Jacobs, *Incidents in the Life of a Slave Girl* (New York: Oxford University Press, 1988), 118

10. Fox-Genovese, *Within the Plantation Household*, 219.

11. bell hooks, *Ain't I A Woman: Black Women and Feminism* (Boston: South End Press, 1981), 55–57. On Reconstruction see W. E. B. Du Bois, *Black Reconstruction in America 1860–1880* (New York: Atheneum, 1962).

12. Mercer, "Black Hair/Black Style," 248.

13. Eliza Potter, *A Hairdresser's Experience in High Life* (New York: Oxford University Press, 1991).

14. Fox-Genovese, *Within the Plantation Household*, 216–18.

15. W. E. B. Du Bois, *The Philadelphia Negro: A Social Study* (New York: Noble Offset Printers, 1967), 116.

16. Interview with Mrs. Grace Garnett-Abney, 28 June 1941, in the "The Negro in Illinois—Beauty Parlors," Work Projects Administration, Illinois Writers' Project, Vivian G. Harsh Research Collection of Afro-American History and Literature, The Carter G. Woodson Regional Library, Chicago, Ill.

17. Joyner, interview with Flug.

18. See, for example, Ethel Erickson, "Employment Conditions in Beauty Shops: A Study of Four Cities," *The Bulletin of the Women's Bureau*, no. 133, 1935.

19. St. Clair Drake and Horace R. Cayton, *Black Metropolis: A Study of Negro Life in a Northern City* (New York: Harcourt, Brace and

Company, 1945), 460. On Jim Crow see C. Vann Woodward, *The Strange Career of Jim Crow*, 3d rev. ed. (New York: Oxford University Press, 1974).

20. Lizabeth Cohen, *Making a New Deal: Industrial Workers in Chicago, 1919–1939* (Cambridge: Cambridge University Press, 1990), 148–49. See also Teresa L. Amott and Julie A. Matthaei, *Race, Gender, and Work: A Multicultural Economic History of Women in the United States* (Boston: South End Press, 1991), 150–51. On the idea of a separate black economy see also Alan H. Spear, *Black Chicago: The Making of a Negro Ghetto, 1890–1920* (Chicago: University of Chicago Press, 1967).

21. Joyner, interview with Flug.

22. Bundles, *Walker*, 63–64.

23. "Biography of Annie Malone," Box 262, Folder 6, Claude A. Barnett Collection, 1889–1967, (hereafter cited CBC) Chicago Historical Society Manuscripts Collection, Chicago, Ill.

24. Nathan E. Jacobs, ed., *NHCA's Golden Years* (Western Publishing Company, 1970), 15.

25. Memorandum From Labor Advisory Board to Deputy Administrator regarding "Code for Beauty Shop Trade—Negro Beauty Shops," 23 February 1934, Box 6094, Folder "File 22 Reports, Studies, and Surveys," Records of the National Recovery Administration (hereafter cited RNRA), Record Group 9, National Archives, Washington, D.C.

26. Jacqueline Jones, *Labor of Love, Labor of Sorrow: Black Women, Work and the Family, From Slavery to the Present* (New York: Vintage Books, 1985), 164.

27. Elizabeth Clark-Lewis, *Living In, Living Out: African American Domestics and the Great Migration* (Washington, D.C.: Smithsonian Institution Press, 1994). See, for example, chapter 4.

28. Bundles, *Walker*, 27

29. Joyner, interview with Flug.

30. Quote from Bundles, *Walker*, 63–64.

31. Amott and Mathaei, *Race, Gender, and Work*, 165, 167–68.

32. Other ethnic groups found hairdressing a means to escape the confines of service work. See, for example, Judy Yung, *Unbound Feet: A Social History of Chinese Women in San Francisco* (Berkeley: University of California Press, 1995), 135.

33. Clark-Lewis, *Living In, Living Out*, 168–69. On domestic service see

also Phyllis Palmer, *Domesticity and Dirt: Housewives and Domestic Servants in the United States, 1920–1945* (Philadelphia: Temple University Press, 1989); Faye E. Dudden, *Serving Women: Household Service in Nineteenth-Century America* (Middleton, Conn.: Wesleyan University Press, 1983).

34. Amott and Matthaei, *Race, Gender, and Work,* 161.

35. Eliot Wigginton, *Refuse to Stand Silently By: An Oral History of Grass Roots Social Activism in America, 1921–1964* (New York: Doubleday Dell, 1991), 180.

36. Evelyn Brooks Higginbotham, *Righteous Discontent: The Women's Movement in the Black Baptist Church, 1880–1920* (Cambridge: Harvard University Press, 1993) 192–93. See also Glenda Elizabeth Gilmore, *Gender and Jim Crow: Women and the Politics of White Supremacy in North Carolina, 1896–1920* (Chapel Hill: The University of North Carolina Press, 1996); Kevin Gaines, *Uplifting the Race: Black Leadership, Politics, and Culture in the Twentieth Century* (Chapel Hill: University of North Carolina Poro College," Chicago Historical Society.

37. Brochure for Annie Malone's "Poro College," Chicago Historical Society.

38. "Pioneers New Important Field," Box 262, Folder 6, CBC.

39. "Personal History of Annie M. Malone," Chicago Historical Society.

40. Peiss, "Making Faces," 388.

41. Rooks, *Hair Raising,* 80–81.

42. Ibid., 63–64.

43. Bundles, *Walker,* 67.

44. Ibid., 80–84, 99–100.

45. "Personal History of Annie M. Turnbo Malone."

46. See advertisement and brief history of Madam Sara S. Washington, Box 261, Folder 7, CBC.

47. See Peiss, *Hope in a Jar;* 5, 67–79; Gwendolyn Robinson, "Class, Race and Gender: A Transcultural, Theoretical and Sociohistorical Analysis of Cosmetic Institutions and Practices to 1920" (Ph.D. diss., University of Illinois at Chicago, 1984).

48. Jacobs, *NHCA's Golden Years,* 6.

49. Emile Beauvais quoted in "Beauty Shop Wants Own Code," National Recovery Administration, 24 August 1933, Box 6094, Folder "File 22 Reports, Studies, and Surveys," RNRA.

50. See, for example, "A Revolutionist Dies," *Life*, 5 February 1951, Box 560, under "Permanent Wave" in the Peter Tamony Collection, Western Historical Manuscripts Collection, Columbia, Missouri.

51. Ida Connolly, *Beauty Operator on Broadway* (Fresno, California: Academy Library Guild, 1954), 47.

52. "Curling Iron Caused Much Consternation," *News Press/ Gazette* (St. Joseph, Mo.), 8 December 1990.

53. Elizabeth Ewen, *Immigrant Women in the Land of Dollars: Life and Culture on the Lower East Side, 1890–1925* (New York: Monthly Review Press, 1985), 33. On immigrant women see also Sydney Stahl Weinberg, *The World of Our Mothers: The Lives of Jewish Immigrant Women* (Chapel Hill: University of North Carolina Press, 1988); Virginia Yans Mclaughlin, *Family and Community: Italian Immigrants in Buffalo, 1880–1930* (Urbana: University of Illinois Press, 1982).

54. Interview with Rose Tellerino (TEL-26), Italians In Chicago, Oral History Project, Chicago Historical Society, Chicago, Illinois, 3.

55. Connolly, *Beauty Operator on Broadway*, 45.

56. Banner, *American Beauty*, 271–72.

57. Jacobs, *NHCA's Golden Years*, 15.

58. Connolly, *Beauty Operator on Broadway*, 45.

59. Jacobs, *NHCA's Golden Years*, 18.

60. Emile Beauvais quoted in "Beauty Shop Wants Own Code," National Recovery Administration, 24 August 1933, Box 6094; Folder "File 22 Reports, Studies, and Surveys," RNRA.

61. Jacobs, *NHCA's Golden Years,* 6; Mark Sullivan,*Our Times, The United States 1900–1925,* and *The Turn of the Century, 1900–1904,* 393–95, in Peter Tamony Collection, Box 97, under "Bobbed Hair."

62. Jacobs, *NHCA's Golden Years*, 5–6.

63. Connolly, *Beauty Operator on Broadway*, 47, 66.

64. Adam Langer, "You Know, I'm 95 and I Know What I'm Talking About," *Chicago Tribune*, 11 September 1992.

65. Peiss, *Hope in a Jar*, 72.

66. Connolly, *Beauty Operator on Broadway*, 69–70.

67. Ibid.

68. See, for example, "A Revolutionist Dies," *Life*, 5 February 1951, in Peter Tamony Collection, Box 560, under "Permanent Wave."

69. Connolly, *Beauty Operator on Broadway*, 77–78; Peiss, *Hope in a Jar*, 78.

70. Gamber, *The Female Economy*, 61. Beauty shops also provided a chance for entrepreneurship much like dressmaking and millinery trades in the nineteenth and early twentieth century, as will be discussed.

71. Connolly, *Beauty Operator on Broadway, 30, 35, 45.*

72. On time management and scientific management see David Montgomery, *Workers' Control in America: Studies in the History of Work, Technology, and Labor Struggles* (Cambridge: Cambridge University Press, 1979); Harry Braverman, *Labor and Monopoly Capital: The Degradation of Work in the Twentieth Century* (New York: Monthly Review Press, 1974).

73. Connolly, *Beauty Operator on Broadway*, 12, 30, 39, 45, 47.

74. Amott and Matthaei, *Race, Gender, and Work*, 127.

75. Emile Beauvais is quoted in "Beauty Shop Wants Own Code," National Recovery Administration, 24 August 1933, Box 6094, Folder "File 22 Reports, Studies, and Surveys," RNRA.

76. Connolly, *Beauty Operator on Broadway*, 62. Other important forms of work that allowed women to combine household chores and paid work included boarding and homework. On homework see Eileen Boris and Cynthia R. Daniels eds., *Homework: Historical and Contemporary Perspectives on Paid Labor at Home* (Urbana: University of Illinois Press, 1989). On boarding see Tamara K. Hareven and John Modell, "Urbanization and the Malleable Household: An Examination of Boarding and Lodging in American Families," *Journal of Marriage and the Family*, 35 (August 1973). On the lifecycle and the beauty ritual see Frida Kerner Furman, *Facing the Mirror: Older Women and Beauty Shop Culture* (New York: Routledge, 1997).

77. Connolly, *Beauty Operator on Broadway*, 50, 34. On "putting on style" see Peiss, *Cheap Amusements*, 57–87.

78. Peiss, *Cheap Amusements*, 42–43.

79. Connolly, *Beauty Operator on Broadway*, 25, 35.

80. Porter Benson, *Counter Cultures*, chapter 3.

81. Connolly, *Beauty Operator on Broadway*, 34. On the rise of dance halls see Peiss, *Cheap Amusements*; 88–114; David Nasaw, *Going Out: The Rise and Fall of Public Amusements* (New York: Basic Books, 1993).

82. Ewen, *Immigrant Women in the Land of Dollars*, 25.

83. "Study of a Family," Box 93, Folder "Family in America, 1938–

1939," Leonard Covello Papers, Balch Institute for Ethnic Studies, Philadelphia, Pennsylvania, 8–9. On the tension between Mexican immigrants and their children see Vicki L. Ruiz, "The Flapper and the Chaperone: Historical Memory among Mexican-American Women," in Donna Gabaccia ed., *Seeking Common Ground: Multidisciplinary Studies of Immigrant Women in the United States* (Connecticut: Greenwood Press, 1992).

84. Connolly, *Beauty Operator on Broadway*, 69

85. Bill Severn, *The Long and Short of It: Five Thousand Years of Fun and Fury over Hair* (New York; David McCay, 1971), 121–22.

86. John D'Emilio and Estelle B. Freedman, *Intimate Matters: A History of Sexuality in America* (New York: Harper and Row, 1988), 241.

87. Christina Simmons, "Companionate Marriage and the Lesbian Threat," *Frontiers* 4, no. 3 (1979), 54–59. On the "new woman" see also Christina Simmons, "Modern Sexuality and the Myth of Victorian Repression," in Kathy Peiss and Christina Simmons, ed., *Passion and Power: Sexuality in History* (Philadelphia: Temple University Press, 1989), 157–77.

88. Carroll Smith-Rosenberg, "Discourses of Sexuality and Subjectivity: The New Woman 1870–1936," in Martin Dubermann et al., *Hidden From History: Reclaiming the Gay and Lesbian Past* (New York: Meridian, 1990), 269.

89. Severn, *The Long and Short of It*, 121–22.

90. Excerpt from Mark Sullivan, *Our Times*, in Peter Tamony Collection, Box 97, under "Bobbed Hair."

91. Albert Howard Wilson, "The Influence of Women's Work on the Barber Business," *The Journeyman Barber*, November 1927, 532–33.

92. Wilson, "The Influence of Women's Work."

93. David Cohn, *A History of American Morals and Manner as Seen through the Sears, Roebuck Catalogs, 1905 to the Present*, 325, in Peter Tamony Collection, Box 97 under "Bobbed Hair."

94. Excerpt from Mark Sullivan, *Our Times*, in Peter Tamony Collection, Box 97, under "Bobbed Hair."

95. Ibid.

96. "Rambling Through Clippins," *The Journeyman Barber*, December 1927, 595. For a discussion of male culture in saloons see Jon Kingsdale, "The Poor Man's Club" in *The American Man*, ed. Eliz-

abeth Pleck and Joseph Pleck (Englewood Cliffs, N.J.: Prentice Hall, 1980): 255–83; Norman H. Clark, *Deliver Us From Evil: An Interpretation of American Prohibition* (New York: W. W. Norton, 1976), 1.

97. "Rambling Through Clippins," *The Journeyman Barber*, December 1927, 595.

98. "Editorial," *The American Hairdresser*, February 1920, 1.

99. "Rambling Through Clippings," *The Journeyman Barber*, April 1929, 99.

100. Wilson, "The Influence of Women's Work," 532–33.

101. C. Vann Woodward, *The Strange Career of Jim Crow*, 116.

102. Jones, *Labor of Love, Labor of Sorrow*, 161.

103. Thomas Kessner, *The Golden Door: Italian and Jewish Immigrant Mobility in New York, 1880–1915* (New York: Oxford University Press, 1977) 33. On the "inbetween" racial status of Italians see Robert Orsi, "The Religious Boundaries of an Inbetween People: Street Feste and the Problem of the Dark-Skinned 'Other' in Italian Harlem, 1920–1990," *American Quarterly*, 44 (Sept. 1992): 313–47.

104. "Males Invading Beauty Parlors for Permanents," Associated Press, Omaha, Nebraska in Women's Bureau, Bulletins, 1918–1963, Record Group 86, "Beauty Shops," Box 241, Folder "Beauty Shops Data," National Archives, Washington, D.C. See also "Modern Barber Shop A Beauty Dispensary," *The Journeyman Barber,* March 1929, 49.

105. Connolly, *Beauty Operator on Broadway*, 48.

106. Ibid., 72.

107. "Excerpts From Diaries of Delinquents," Institute For Juvenile Research, Box 7, Folder 6, Chicago Historical Society, Chicago, Illinois, 11–12.

108. Blonde hair became popular after a burlesque troupe from Britain toured the United States. According to Banner, the members of the troupe "peroxided their hair and became blonde. For half a century, brown hair had been the favored color. Now light blonde hair became the vogue." See Banner, *American Beauty*, 121; Peiss, *Hope in a Jar*, 39, 48.

109. Gaetano De Filippis, "Social Life in an Immigrant Community," Box 130, Folder 2, Ernest Burgess Papers, University of Chicago, Chicago, Ill., 8.

110. Cobble, *Dishing It Out*, 22.

111. Wendy Cooper, *Hair: Sex, Society, Symbolism* (New York: Stein and Day, 1971), 76–77.

112. Charles Berg, *The Unconscious Significance of Hair* (Leicester: Blackfriars Press, 1951), 34.

113. Harvey Green, *Fit for America: Health, Fitness, Sport and American Society* (Baltimore: Johns Hopkins University Press, 1986), 253. On immigration restriction and nativism see John Higham, *Strangers in the Land: Patterns of American Nativism* (New Brunswick: Rutgers University Press, 1955); Dale T. Knobel, *America for the Americans: The Nativist Movement in the United States* (New York: Twayne Publishers, 1996).

114. Cooper, *Hair: Sex, Society, Symbolism*, 76–77.

115. Ibid., 76.

116. Anzia Yezierska, *Bread Givers* (New York: Persea Books, 1975), 4. For a discussion of female beauty and intelligence in the nineteenth century see Banner, *American Beauty*, 124.

117. bell hooks, *Black Looks: Race and Representation* (Boston: South End Press, 1992), 21–22.

118. Kevin J. Mumford, *Interzones: Black/White Sex Districts in Chicago and New York in the Early Twentieth Century* (New York: Columbia University Press, 1997), xviii, 134–35, 162–67. On the Great Migration see also James R. Grossman, *Land of Hope: Chicago, Black Southerners, and the Great Migration* (Chicago: University of Chicago Press, 1989).

119. For a discussion of racial identity and blackface see David Roediger, *Wages of Whiteness: Race and the Making of the American Working Class* (New York: Verso, 1991); Eric Lott, *Love and Theft: Blackface Minstrelsy and the American Working Class* (New York: Oxford University Press, 1993).

Notes to Chapter 2

1. Lucille Miller, n.d., Box 6088, Folder "Classification (N-Q)," RNRA.

2. Ibid.

3. National Industrial Recovery Administration, Hearing on Code of Fair Practices and Competition, 20 February 1934, 55–57, Box 227, Folder "Transcripts of Hearings 1933–1935," RNRA.

4. National Recovery Administration Memorandum, Form 17A, From

Labor Advisory Board to Deputy Administrator Olsen, 23 February 1934, Box 6094, Folder "File 22 Reports, Studies and Surveys," RNRA.

5. National Industrial Recovery Administration, Hearing on Code of Fair Practices and Competition, 20 February 1934, 52, 56–57, Box 227, Folder "Transcripts of Hearings, 1933–1935," RNRA.

6. See, for example, Porter Benson, *Counter Cultures*; Cobble, *Dishing it Out*; and Gamber, *The Female Economy*, 106.

7. On the rise of professional and white-collar work see Amott and Matthaei, *Race, Gender, and Work*, 122–23, 127; Alice Kessler-Harris, *Out to Work: A History of Wage Earning Women in the United States* (New York: Oxford University Press, 1982), 114–17; Sharon Hartman Strom, *Beyond the Typewriter: Gender, Class, and the Origins of Modern American Office Work, 1900–1930* (Urbana: University of Illinois Press, 1992).

8. National Industrial Recovery Administration, Hearing on Code of Fair Practices and Competition, 20 February 1934, 55, Box 227, Folder "Transcripts of Hearings 1933–1935," RNRA.

9. Box 6093, *Investigate Burnham's . . . Before Enrolling in Any Beauty School*, Folder 21, "Publications," RNRA

10. Ibid.

11. *The Wilfred System of Hair and Beauty Culture*, Box 6093, Folder 21, "Publications," RNRA.

12. *Employment Opportunities in Beauty Shops of New York City*, State of New York, Department of Labor, Division of Women in Industry, 1931, 37, and or a discussion of "all-round girls" and the types of work in beauty shops, see also *Employment Opportunities in Beauty Shops*, 13.

13. *Investigate Burnham's . . . Before Enrolling in any Beauty School*, Box 6093, Folder 21, "Publications," RNRA.

14. *Employment Opportunities in Beauty Shops of New York City*, 37.

15. Ibid.

16. *The Wilfred System of Hair and Beauty Culture*, Box 6093, Folder 21, RNRA.

17. *Investigate Burnham's . . . Before Enrolling in Any Beauty School*, Box 6093, Folder 21, RNRA.

18. Banner, *American Beauty*, 216.

19. Elizabeth Gideon, North Platte Nebraska, 9 March 1934, Box 6090, Folder 11 "(E-G)," RNRA.

20. *Employment Opportunities in Beauty Shops of New York City*, 35.

21. Ibid., 38.

22. Emile Beauvais, quoted in "Beauty Shops Want Own Code," 24 August 1933, National Recovery Administration, Box 6094, Folder "File 22, Reports, Studies, and Surveys," RNRA.

23. Daisy Schwartz, New York, n.d., Box 6089, Folder 11, "General (A-B)," RNRA.

24. Elizabeth Gideon, North Platte, Nebraska, 9 March 1934, Box 6090, Folder 11, "(E-G)," RNRA.

25. Mabel English Sanders, Savanna, Georgia, n.d., Box 6090, Folder 11, "(E-G)," RNRA.

26. Betty Jean, Mansfield, Ohio, 16 September 1933, Box 6087, Folder 4, "Classification A-Z," RNRA.

27. *Employment Opportunities in Beauty Shops of New York City*, 18–19.

28. National Industrial Recovery Administration, Hearing on Code of Fair Practices and Competition, 20 February 1934, 43–44, Box 227, Folder "Transcripts of Hearings 1933–1935," RNRA.

29. Interview with Louise Long, December 1994. All the oral history interviews were conducted by the author unless otherwise noted and all the interviewees were given pseudonyms.

30. Interview with Mrs. Leland (Everett) Hall, 20–21, Oral History Collection, University Archives, Sangamon State University, Springfield, Illinois.

31. Horace J. Smith, "Do You Know the Laws Governing Your Profession!" *The American Hairdresser*, December 1931, 48–49, 68–69.

32. Investigators found one "school for Negro Operators," which demanded students be at least eighteen years of age and have completed the eighth grade. Another exception with regards to education were public schools which required a minimum education, usually the eighth grade or the equivalent of junior high school work. See *Employment Opportunities in Beauty Shops of New York City*, 35.

33. Ibid., 35–36.

34. Ibid., 19–20, 36.

35. The price for a press and shampoo before the Depression was usually $1.50 or $2.00. By 1933, the average price dropped to one dollar. See Erickson, *Employment Conditions in Beauty Shops*, 38–40.

36. Women's Bureau, Unpublished Studies and Materials, 1919–1972, Box 241, Folder "Summary of Negro Shops."

37. *Employment Opportunities in Beauty Shops of New York City*, 11, 22.
38. "Business Hints From Eastern Shops," *The American Hairdresser*, February 1929, 104.
39. Lucille Miller, n.d., Box 6088, Folder "Classification N-Q," RNRA.
40. "Do Your Operator's Uniforms and Personal Appearance Inspire the Confidence of Your Clients?," *The American Hairdresser*, October, 1931, 68–69. On uniforms see Clark-Lewis, *Living In, Living Out*, 113–17, 159–61.
41. Murray Kane, Cincinnati, Ohio, 17 January 1934, Box 6088, Folder 6 "Complaints," RNRA.
42. Vice President of the "NIRA" Beauty Culture Code, Association of Illinois, Chicago, Ill., 22 September 1933, Box 6087, Folder 4 "Classification A-Z," RNRA.
43. "Beauty Shop Wants Own Code." The expression "Bath-room beauty shop" is used by Emile Beauvais, Box 6094, Folder "File 22, Reports, Studies, and Surveys," RNRA.
44. *Employment Opportunities in Beauty Shops of New York City*, 11, 18, 27.
45. Jones, *Labor of Love, Labor of Sorrow*, 214.
46. Erickson, *Employment Conditions in Beauty Shops*, 37.
47. Interviews and newspaper clippings about Mrs. Emma Shelton, Winona Historical Society, Winona, Minnesota.
48. Erickson, *Employment Conditions in Beauty Shops*, 38–39.
49. Connolly, *Beauty Operator on Broadway*, 95–96. For an overview of women during the Depression see Susan Ware, *Holding Their Own: American Women in the 1930s* (Boston: Twayne Publishers, 1982).
50. Connolly, *Beauty Operator on Broadway*, 94, 96.
51. Ibid., 48.
52. Grace Voight, "Tackling Tough Customers With Tact," *The Beautician*, July 1924, 14–16. Wendy Gamber notes that in certain occupations like dressmaking, the worker was expected to do more than create a final product. Like a new hair style, a new dress was an assertion of identity. Customers' expectations made them especially difficult to please in such service industries. See Gamber, *The Female Economy*, 113.
53. Connolly, *Beauty Operator on Broadway*, 66.
54. Mary Triella, Dover, New Jersey, 2 October 1938, Box 6088, Folder 4, "Classification R-Z," RNRA.
55. Voight, "Tackling Tough Customers With Tact."

56. Arlie Russell Hochschild, *The Managed Heart: Commercialization of Human Feeling* (Berkeley: University of California Press, 1983), 3–23, 162–84.

57. Interview with Betty Saunders on "Say It With Words" KFRC-San Francisco Radio Program, 2 August 1938, in Peter Tamony Collection, Box 63 under "Beauty Parlor." On language see also Marcus Rediker, *Between the Devil and the Deep Blue Sea: Merchant Seamen, Pirates, and the Anglo-American Maritime World, 1700–1750* (Cambridge: Cambridge University Press, 1987), 53, 211, 162–69. See also Sterling Stuckey, *Going Through The Storm: The Influence of African American Art in History* (New York: Oxford University Press, 1994), 3–18; Roediger, *Wages of Whiteness*, 43–64.

58. Madame Louise, "Trouble Corner," *The American Hairdresser*, July 1932, 50.

59. Madame Louise, "Trouble Corner," *The American Hairdresser*, July 1938, 47.

60. Dr. Morris M. Estrin, "Beautician's Eczema?" *The American Hairdresser*, February 1933, 38–39.

61. Survey of Negro Beauty Shops in the District of Columbia, under "Hazards," Box 130, Folder "Negro Beauty Shops in the District of Columbia 1939, "The Women's Bureau Unpublished Studies and Materials 1919–1972. Beauticians still face a number of health hazards. See Patricia McCormack, "Beauticians Found Facing Cancer Risk," *Los Angeles Times*, 10 January 1985.

62. *Short Cuts for The Beauty Shop* (Pasadena: Chap Book Press, 1933), 3, 21.

63. National Industrial Recovery Administration, Hearing on Code of Fair Practices and Competition, 20 February 1934, 55–57, Box 227, Folder "Transcripts of Hearings 1933–1935," RNRA, 51.

64. *Employment Opportunities in Beauty Shops of New York City*, 12, 23, 24.

65. "Legends of Cosmetology: Lydia Adams—Cosmetologist, Teacher, Businessperson, Amateur Golfer," *Shoptalk*, Winter 1984, 87–88.

66. Erickson, *Employment Conditions in Beauty Shops*, 42.

67. *Employment Opportunities in Beauty Shops of New York City*, 12.

68. Helen Milner, "Air-Conditioning Makes Women Have More Work Done," *The American Hairdresser*, June 1935, 66.

69. Florence Raberge, "Defeat the Hot Weather 'Bugaboo,'" *The American Hairdresser*, July 1936, 32–33.

70. "Five Shops in One St. Louis Block," *The American Hairdresser*, October 1938, 93.

71. Ibid.

72. Connolly, *Beauty Operator on Broadway*, 80.

73. Raberge, "Defeat the Hot Weather 'Bugaboo,'" 32–33.

74. Doly Phillips Hanline, "Ohio Beauticians Renew Fight to Bring Industry Under State Minimum Wage Law," *The Journeyman Barber Hairdresser and Cosmetologist*, October 1939, 10.

75. Report of the Industrial Commissioner to the Beauty Shop Minimum Wage Board, State of New York, Department of Labor, Division of Women in Industry and Minimum Wage, March 1938, 6.

76. Report of the Industrial Commissioner to the Beauty Shop Minimum Wage Board, 3–4.

77. Ibid., 9.

78. Marian Varley, New York City, 23 November 1933, Box 6088, Folder 4 "Classification (R-Z)," RNRA.

79. *Employment Opportunities in Beauty Shops of New York City*, 12.

80. Women's Bureau findings summarized in "Working Conditions in Beauty Shops Described in Department of Labor Bulletin," *The Journeyman Barber*, July 1935, 26.

81. *Employment Opportunities in Beauty Shops of New York City*, 13, 16.

82. Albert Howard Wilson, "The Influence of Women's Work On The Barber Business," *The Journeyman Barber*, November 1927, "Five Shops in One St. Louis Block," *The American Hairdresser*, October 1938, 93.

83. James C. Shanessy, "Women Beauty Workers In Need of Organization," *The Journeyman Barber*, December 1927, 597.

84. Jacobs, *Golden Years*, 10; "Beauticians, Organize and Educate," *The Journeyman Barber Hairdresser and Cosmetologist*, May 1937, 21.

85. James C. Shanessy, "Women Beauty Workers In Need of Organization," *The Journeyman Barber*, December 1927, 597.

86. Saide Reisch to Gail Wilson, 22 August 1927, Papers of the National Women's Trade Union League Papers and Its Principal Leaders, Collection II, National Women's Trade Union League Papers, Schlesinger Library, on microfilm under "Industries-Beauty Parlor," The Manuscript Division, Library of Congress, Washington, D.C.

87. For examples of successful organization efforts see the following: Adelaide Fielding, "Beauty Shop Workers Organizing Rapidly in

Los Angeles and Vicinity," *The Journeyman Barber Hairdresser and Cosmetologist*, August 1937, 5; "Beauticians Learn Value of Unionism," *The Journeyman Barber Hairdresser and Cosmetologist*, August 1937, 21; "Why the Public Should Patronize Union Beauticians, *The Journeyman Barber Hairdresser and Cosmetologist*, June 1939, 26; Dolly Phillips Hanline, "Ohio Beauticians Renew Fight to Bring Industry Under State Minimum Wage Law," *The Journeyman Barber Hairdresser and Cosmetologist*, October 1939, 10.

88. Joseph De Silvis, "This Help Problem," *The National Beauty Shop*, May 1929, 44, 52.

89. A. L. Barber, "Do Your Operators Attract or Drive Away Patrons?" *The American Hairdresser*, August 1928, 72.

90. Porter Benson, *Counter Cultures*, 259.

91. Hazel Koslay, "Who Owns Your Shop . . . You or Your Operators?" *The American Hairdresser*, November 1939, 31.

92. Ibid.

93. Letter to Mr. Harry Spiro, President, New York Hairdressers and Cosmetologists Association, n.d., Box 6088, Folder "Classification N-Q," RNRA. For similar examples of worker resistance see Tera W. Hunter, *To 'Joy My Freedom: Southern Black Women's Lives and Labors after the Civil War* (Cambridge: Harvard University Press, 1997.)

94. *Employment Opportunities in Beauty Shops of New York City*, 13.

Notes to Chapter 3

1. Laura E. Wernsman, Eureka, Illinois, 9 January 1934, Box 6089, Folder 10, "Explanation," RNRA.

2. Ellis W. Hawley, *The New Deal and the Problem of Monopoly: A Study in Economic Ambivalence* (Princeton, New Jersey: Princeton University Press, 1966), 53–54.

3. Jacobs, *NHCA's Golden Years*, 8–11. On how the breakdown of certain institutions can affect community life see Ardis Cameron, *Radicals of the Worst Sort: Laboring Women in Lawrence, Massachusetts, 1860–1912* (Urbana: University of Illinois Press, 1993).

4. F. A. Hood of Margaret Hood's Beauty Salon, Great Falls Montana, 21 February 1934, Box 6088, Folder 6, "Complaints," RNRA.

5. See "Beauty Shops Want Own Code," 24 August 1933, Box 6094, Folder "File 22, Reports, Studies, and Surveys," RNRA.

6. "Beauty Shops Want Own Code." According to the NHCA report, "the census department has not broken down the classification of 'barbers, hairdressers, and manicurists' except by sexes, and therefore it is impossible to know just how many of each there are. The total of both increased from 216,211 in 1920 to 374,290 in 1930. Since beauty shop operators are almost universally women, we believe the 'female enumerative' gives a good index of the flood of newcomers, for the 1920 census show 33,246 as against 113,194."

7. "'Young, Slim and Nice Looking—' How?" *Life and Labor Bulletin*, National Women's Trade Union League of America, 5, no. 9, October 1927.

8. "'Young, Slim and Nice Looking—' How?"

9. Elizabeth Christman, Secretary-Treasurer, to The Journeyman Barbers' International Union of America, 24 June 1934, National Women's Trade Union League of America, Papers of the WTUL, 3.

10. "First Permanent Made Her a Hot Head," *News-Press/Gazette* (St. Joseph, Mo.), 28 December 1990.

11. "Permanently Put Off by Permanents," *News-Press/Gazette* (St. Joseph, Mo.), 28 December 1990.

12. "Early Permanent Heavy on the Head," *News-Press/Gazette* (St. Joseph, Mo.), 28 December 1990.

13. "Use of Hot Comb Led to Hair-Raising Experience," *News-Press/Gazette* (St. Joseph, Mo.), 28 December 1990.

14. Marian Varley to Mr. Emile Martin, President of the New York State Hairdressers Association, 23 November 1933, Box 6088, Folder 4, "Classification (R-Z)," RNRA.

15. Francis M. Jones, Burlington, Iowa, 28 February 1934, Box 6090, Folder 11 "General (E-G)," RNRA.

16. National Industrial Recovery Administration, Hearing on Code of Fair Practices and Competition, 20 February 1934, Box 227, Folder "Transcripts of Hearings 1933–1935," RNRA, 175–78.

17. Jacobs, *NHCA's Golden Years*, 15.

18. National Industrial Recovery Administration, Hearing on Code of Fair Practices and Competition, 20 February 1934, Box 227, Folder "Transcripts of Hearings 1933–1935," RNRA, 179.

19. National Industrial Recovery Administration, Hearing on Code of

Fair Practices and Competition, 20 February 1934, Box 227, Folder "Transcripts of Hearings 1933–1935," RNRA, 180, 183–85.

20. Daisy Schwartz, General (A-B), RNRA.

21. National Industrial Recovery Administration, Hearing on Code of Fair Practices and Competition, 20 February 1934, Box 227, Folder "Transcripts of Hearings 1933–1935," RNRA, 119.

22. National Industrial Recovery Administration, Hearing on Code of Fair Practices and Competition, 20 February 1934, Box 227, Folder "Transcripts of Hearings 1933–1935," RNRA, 52–53.

23. Jean Gray, Chicago, Illinois, 14 January 1934, Box 6091, Folder 16, "Labor," RNRA.

24. Mrs. J. H. Riggan, Texas Association of Accredited Beauty Culturists, Inc., 28 November 1933, Box 6088, Folder 6, "Complaints," RNRA.

25. Carol B. Hepburn, Hammonton, New Jersey, 25 September 1933, Box 6094, Folder 24, "Selling Below Cost," RNRA.

26. Hazel Bartholf, 10 October 1933 Box 6087, Folder 4, "Classification (A-G)," RNRA.

27. Ibid.

28. A. C. Patch, Topeka, Kansas, 28 July 1933, Box 6090, Folder 11 "General (O-S)," RNRA.

29. National Industrial Recovery Administration, Hearing on Code of Fair Practices and Competition, 20 February 1934, Box 227, Folder "Transcripts of Hearings 1933–1935," RNRA, 185. For a discussion of the popular condemnation of married women who engaged in wage work during the Depression see Alice Kessler-Harris, *Out to Work*, 253–56.

30. Josephine Nichols, New Brunswick, New Jersey, 3 August 1934, Box 6089, Folder, "General (A-B)," RNRA.

31. Thomas S. Hammond, August 1933, Box 6090, Folder 11, "General (H-K)," RNRA.

32. Grace Brost, Sunbury, Pennsylvania, 30 November 1933, Box 6089, Folder 10, "Explanations," RNRA.

33. Charles J. Kutill, "Now Is The Time," *Modern Beauty Shop*, September 1933, Box 6087, Folder 4, "Classification (A-Z)," RNRA.

34. Anne Buchanan, Norton, Virginia, 8 September 1933, Box 6091, Folder 16, "Labor," RNRA.

35. Agnes Plant, Sauk Centre, Minnesota, 19 August 1933, Box 6090, Folder 11, "General (O-S)," RNRA.

36. E. P. Thompson, *The Making of the English Working Class* (New York: Vintage, 1966), 63.

37. Mrs. Ines Conner, Newton, Kansas, 12 September 1933, Box 6090, Folder "(C-D)," RNRA.

38. Mrs. R. A. Collins, Athens, Georgia, 23 August 1933, Box 6087, Folder 4, "Classification (A-G)," RNRA.

39. "Are You Overlooking the Prolific Business of the RURAL WOMAN?," *The American Hairdresser*, July 1932, 36.

40. Interview with Angela Roberts, November 1994, Columbia, Missouri.

41. "Walk a Mile, or 10, for a Permanent," *News-Press/Gazette* (St. Joseph, MO), 28 December 1990. On consumption and the rural woman see Mary Neth, *Preserving the Family Farm: Women, Community, and the Foundations of Agribusiness in the Midwest, 1900–1940* (Baltimore: Johns Hopkins University Press, 1995), 187–213.

42. James M. Kefford, New York, 4 November 1933, Box 6090, Folder 11, "General (C-D)," RNRA.

43. Daisy Brown, Tampa, Florida, n.d., Box 6094, Folder 24, "Selling Below Cost," RNRA.

44. Annabell Criswell, Dallas, Texas, 11 August 1933, Box 6089, Folder 10, "Explanations," RNRA.

45. Elenora Christiansen, Savannah, Georgia, 22 August 1933, Box 6090, Folder 11, "General (C-D)," RNRA.

46. Jane Brown, Kansas City, Missouri, 22 August 1932, Box 6087, Folder 4, "Classification A-G" RNRA.

47. Mrs. R. A. Collins, Athens, Georgia, 23 August 1933, Box 6087, Folder 4, "Classification A-G" RNRA.

48. [Author unknown], letter written to Thomas S. Hammond, August, 1933, Box 6090, Folder 11, "General (H-K)," RNRA.

49. The NRA undermined other small Chicago shopkeepers who found they could not compete with chain stores under new wage and price codes. See, for example, Cohen, *Making a New Deal*, 236–38.

50. Mrs. Leo Farmer, Dallas, Texas, 23 August 1933, Box 6090, Folder 11, "General (E-G)," RNRA.

51. [Author unknown], letter to Mr. Hugh S. Johnson, Indianapolis, Indiana, September 1933, Box 6094, Folder 24, "Selling Below Cost," RNRA.

52. Mrs. Ines Conner, Newton, Kansas, 12 September 1933, Box 6090, Folder 11, "General (C-D)," RNRA.

53. National Industrial Recovery Administration, Hearing on Code of Fair Practices and Competition, 20 February 1934, Box 227, Folder "Transcripts of Hearings 1933–1935," RNRA, 119–20.

54. [Author unknown], letter written to the National Recovery Act Administration, 22 September 1933, Box 6087, Folder 4, "Classification A-Z," RNRA.

55. American Cosmeticians Association, 22 February 1934, Box 6089, Folder 11, "General (A-B)," RNRA.

56. Harold A. Dempsey, Attorney for the American Cosmeticians Association, New Orleans, 5 January 1934, Box 6087, Folder 4, "Classification, (A-G)," RNRA.

57. Catherine J. Danner, Emporium, Pennsylvania, 27 June 1934, Box 6089, Folder 11 "General (A-B)," RNRA.

58. Leta May Johnson, 23 November 1933, Box 6090, Folder 11, "General (H-K), RNRA.

59. William E. Trull, Wichita, Kansas, 25 July 1933, Box 6091, Folder 11, "General P.R.A." RNRA.

60. Jacobs, *NHCA,'s Golden Years*, 19–20.

61. "Wanted a Classification," *The American Hairdresser*, September 1933, 17.

62. In the early twentieth century, millinery trade journals made similar claims that women failed to act in a businesslike manner. See Gamber, *The Female Economy*, 172.

63. Lillian Flyer, "Sanitation (?) as Found in Some Neighborhood Beauty Shops," *The American Hairdresser*, March 1939, 52–53, 73.

64. Ibid.

65. See, for example, Flyer, "Sanitation," and Hazel Koslay, "Who Owns Your Shop . . . You or Your Operators?" *The American Hairdresser*, November 1939, 31.

66. Harold A. Dempsey, Attorney for the American Cosmeticians Association, New Orleans, 5 January 1934, Box 6087, Folder 4, "Classification (A-G)," RNRA.

67. National Industrial Recovery Administration, Hearing on Code of Fair Practices and Competition, 20 February 1934, Box 227, Folder "Transcripts of Hearings 1933–1935," RNRA, 200.

68. Melosh, *"The Physician's Hand,"* 19–20.

69. Manning Marable, *How Capitalism Underdeveloped Black America: Problems in Race, Political Economy, and Society* (Boston: South End Press, 1983), 184.

70. Joe William Trotter, Jr., *Black Milwaukee: The Making of an Indus-*
    trial Proletariat, 1915–1945 (Urbana: University of Illinois Press,
    1985), 9, 12.
71. Trotter, *Black Milwaukee*, 159; Amott and Matthaei, *Race, Gender,
    and Work*, 127.
72. Mrs. J. H. Riggan, Texas Association of Accredited Beauty Cultur-
    ists, Inc., 28 November 1933, Box 6088, Folder 6, "Complaints,"
    RNRA. These same arguments were made in a letter from Thos D.
    Scott, Texas Association of Accredited Beauty Culturists, Inc. 17
    November 1933, Box 6087, Folder 4, "Classification (A-Z)," RNRA.
73. Virginia Williams, Jacksonville, Florida, 31 October 1935, Box
    6087, Folder "Beauty Shop Trade," RNRA.
74. Mary Tirella, Dover, New Jersey, 2 October 1933, Box 6088, Folder
    4, "Classification (R-Z)," RNRA.
75. Jim's Beauty Studio, Hollywood, 8 August 1933, Box 6090, Folder
    11, "General (H-K)," RNRA.
76. Drake and Cayton, *Black Metropolis*, 218–20. According to Drake
    and Cayton, 72 percent of service occupations in Chicago in 1930
    were filled by foreign-born and African-American laborers.
77. Telegraph from The Chicago and Illinois Hairdressers Association,
    3 August 1933, Box 6087, Folder 4, "Classification (A-G)," RNRA.
78. Drake and Cayton, *Black Metropolis*, 235.
79. Telegraph from The Chicago and Illinois Hairdressers Association,
    3 August 1933, Box 6087, Folder 4, "Classification (A-G)," RNRA.
80. Roediger, *Wages of Whiteness*.
81. W. E. B. Du Bois, *Black Reconstruction in America, 1860–1880* (New
    York: Antheneum Publisher, 1935), 700.

Notes to Chapter 4

1. "Lulline Long: Selling Care and Concern," *Shoptalk*, Spring 1985,
   111.
2. Vernon Scott, "Much (2.7 Billion) Ado About Hairdos," *Pageant*,
   May 1962, 124–30, in Peter Tamony Collection, Box 344, under
   "Hair."
3. Ruth Milkman, *Gender at Work: The Dynamics of Job Segregation
   by Sex during World War II* (Urbana: University of Illinois Press
   1987), 51, 121–22.

4. Hazel Koslay, "Editorial," *The American Hairdresser*, April 1942, 15.

5. Hazel Kozlay, "Editorial," *The American Hairdresser*, March 1943, 21. See also "State Boards Approach Relief of Operator Shortage," *The American Hairdresser*, August 1943, 52–53.

6. Jacobs, *NHCA's Golden Years*, 29.

7. Hazel Kozlay, "Editorial," *The American Hairdresser*, March 1943, 21.

8. Jacobs, *NHCA's Golden Years*, 28.

9. Hazel Koslay, "The Editorial Slant," *The American Hairdresser*, July 1943, 22–23.

10. "Letters to the Editor," *The American Hairdresser*, April 1942, 60.

11. "IN THE NEWS—IN MISSOURI . . . ," *The American Hairdresser*, January 1943, 64–65.

12. "The Ever-Enduring Maude Gadsen," *Shoptalk*, Spring 1986, 100–101.

13. "IN THE NEWS—IN MISSOURI . . . ," *The American Hairdresser*, January 1943, 64–65.

14. Peiss, *Hope in a Jar*, 239.

15. Jacobs, *NHCA's Golden Years*, 28.

16. See, for example, Milkman, *Gender at Work*, 61.

17. Clairol advertisement in *The American Hairdresser*, May 1942, 5.

18. "Use a Patriotic Theme in Your Window," *The American Hairdresser*, January 1942, 52.

19. Jacobs, *NHCA's Golden Years*, 28. On women during World War II see Miriam Frank, Marilyn Ziebarth, and Connie Field, *The Life and Times of Rosie the Riveter: The Story of Three Million Working Women During World War II* (Emeryville, Calif.: Clarity Educational Productions, 1982).

20. "Use a Patriotic Theme in Your Window," *The American Hairdresser*, January 1942, 52.

21. "Styled for War Work," *The American Hairdresser*, April 1942, 22.

22. "IN THE NEWS—IN MISSOURI . . . ," *The American Hairdresser*, January 1943, 64–65. On the history of the WACs see Allan Bérubé, *Coming Out under Fire: The History of Gay Men and Women in World War Two* (New York: Penguin Books, 1991). See also Georgia Clark Sadler, "From Women's Services to Servicewomen," in Francine D'Amico and Laurie Weinstein ed., *Gender Camouflage: Women and the U.S. Military* (New York: New York University Press, 1999).

Notes to Chapter 4

23. Jane Dickson, "Beauty Shop—Army Style," *The American Hair-* 223
    dresser, September 1943, 58, 69.

24. "Beauty Morale for War Plant's 'Victory Girls,'" *The American Hairdresser*, February 1943, 23, 70.

25. On child care issues during World War II see Kessler-Harris, *Out to Work*, 290–95.

26. "Beauty Comes to a War Plant," *The American Hairdresser*, April 1943, 55. See also Peiss, *Hope in a Jar*, 242.

27. Elaine Tyler May, *Homeward Bound: American Families in the Cold War Era* (New York: Basic Books, 1988), 74.

28. Robin D. G. Kelley, *Race Rebels: Culture, Politics, and the Black Working Class* (New York: Free Press, 1994), 163–64.

29. Langer, "You Know, I'm 95 and I Know What I'm Talking About"; "The Marjorie Stewart Joyner Collection: Chronological History of Dr. Marjorie Stewart Joyner," The Chicago Historical Society, Current Collecting Correspondence Collection, under "Joyner."

30. Herbert Shapiro, *White Violence and Black Response: From Reconstruction to Montgomery* (Amherst: University of Massachusetts Press, 1988), 337.

31. See Joyner interview with Flug.

32. Marable, *Race Reform, and Rebellion*, 14, 23.

33. Malanna Carey, "The Smithsonian Salutes a Real Pioneer," *Beauty Classic*, 4, no. 1, 1987, 30–31, 52.

34. Jacobs, *NHCA's Golden Years*, 32–33.

35. Clifford M. Kuhn, Harlon E. Joye, E. Bernard West, *Living Atlanta: An Oral History of the City, 1914–1918* (Athens: University of Georgia Press, 1990), 110.

36. Eliot Wigginton, ed., *Refuse to Stand Silently By: An Oral History of Grass Roots Social Activism in America, 1921–1964* (New York: Doubleday Dell, 1991), 245–46.

37. Aldon D. Morris, *The Origins of the Civil Rights Movement: Back Communities Organizing for Change* (New York: Free Press, 1984), 145–46. On the Civil Rights Movement see also Doug McAdam, *Political Process and the Development of Black Insurgency 1930–1970* (Chicago: University of Chicago Press, 1982).

38. Morris, *The Origins of the Civil Rights Movement*, 139–40.

39. "Memo From the Editorial Staff—The Breck Survey," *The American Hairdresser*, June 1953, 33.

40. "VOGUE Survey Shows High Beauty-Shop Attendance," *The American Hairdresser*, January 1952, 54, 71.

41. "The Shop with Once-A-Week customers,"*The American Hairdresser*, July 1951, 62, 83–84.

42. "Memo From the Editorial Staff—The Breck Survey," *The American Hairdresser*, June 1953, 33. See also *Employment Opportunities for Women in Beauty Service*, U.S. Department of Labor, Women's Bureau Bulletin no. 260, 1956, 2–3.

43. "From the Editorial Staff," *The American Hairdresser*, June 1953, 33.

44. Lillian Blackstone, "My Entire Business is Teens!" *The American Hairdresser*, September 1948, 62, 64, 92. For information on the cosmetic industry's interest in the teenage market see Peiss, *Hope in a Jar*, 246.

45. Elaine Budd, "Your Teen Trade Means More Business," *The American Hairdresser*, August, 1956, 68–69.

46. Beth Bailey, *From Front Porch to Back Seat: Courtship in Twentieth-Century America* (Baltimore: Johns Hopkins University Press, 1988), 50–51, 60–62.

47. Elaine Budd, "Your Teen Trade Means More Business," *The American Hairdresser*, August, 1956, 68–69. On teenage girls in the 1950s see Wini Breines, Y*oung, White, and Miserable: Growing Up Female in the Fifties* (Boston: Beacon Press, 1992).

48. Anne Moody, *Coming of Age in Mississippi* (New York: Dell, 1968), 105–6.

49. Marable, *Race, Rebellion and Reform*, 16–17; Amott and Matthaei, *Race, Gender, and Work*, 173

50. Weems, *Desegregating the Dollar*, 34.

51. *Employment Opportunities for Women in Beauty Service*, 2; Kessler-Harris, *Out to Work*, 300–305.

52. Vernon Scott, "Much ($2.7 Billion) Ado About Hairdos," *Pageant*, May 1962, 124–30, in Peter Tamony Collection, Box 344, under "Hair."

53. "Beauty-The Industry without a Recession," 86–90 *Time*, 16 June 1958, in Peter Tamony Collection, Box 63, under "Beauty Industry."

54. Vernon Scott, "Much ($2.7 Billion) Ado About Hairdos," *Pageant*, May 1962, 124–30, in Peter Tamony Collection, Box 344, under "Hair."

55. See, for example, advertisements in *Ebony*, July 1954, 88, in Peter Tamony Collection, Box 344, under "Hair"; *Ebony* July 1957, 107 in Peter Tamony Collection, Box 344, under "Hair"; *Our World*, July 1954, 9, 75, 81, in Peter Tamony Collection, Box 344, under "Hair."

56. Hazel Koslay, "The Editorial Slant," *The American Hairdresser*, January 1945, 34.

57. Lillian Blackstone, "My Entire Business Is Teens!" *The American Hairdresser*, September 1948, 62, 64, 92.

58. "Beauty—The Industry Without a Recession," *Time*, 16 June 1958, in Peter Tamony Collection Box 63, under "Hair"; second part of quote from "College Girls 'Put on Dog,'" San Francisco State College, 26 June 1952, in Peter Tamony Collection, Box 582, under "Poodle Cut."

59. Scott, "Much (2.7 billion) Ado About Hairdos," *Pageant*, May 1962, 124–30, in Peter Tamony Collection, Box 344, under "Hair."

60. *Employment Opportunities for Women in Beauty Service*, 3–4.

61. Robert R. Hoffman and Herbert S. Rosen, "Two Views on the Shortage of Operators," *The American Hairdresser*, October 1952, 48–49, 73.

62. "Memo from the Editor," *The American Hairdresser*, May 1952, 31.

63. Hoffman and Rosen, "Two Views on the Shortage of Operators," 48–49, 73.

64. Robert Fiance, "Part Four," *The American Hairdresser*, May 1951, 56–57.

65. Robert Fiance, "Time and Motion Study—The First in a New Series," *The American Hairdresser*, February 1951, 62–63. On time management and scientific management see Montgomery, *Workers' Control in America*; Harry Braverman, *Labor and Monopoly Capital*.

66. Hoffman and Rosen, "Two Views on the Shortage of Operator," 48–49, 73.

67. "College Girls 'Put on Dog,'" San Francisco State College, 26 June 1952, in Peter Tamony Collection, Box 582, under "Poodle Cut."

68. Severn, *The Long and Short of It*, 126. Last quote from Inez Robb, "She's Got Beehives in Her Bonnet!" 26 May 1960, *San Francisco Examiner*, in Peter Tamony Collection, Box 345, under "Hair."

69. Brenda Fike, "Retiring Beautician Has Seen Hairstyles Come and Go in Her 55 years of Business," *The Mexico Ledger* (Missouri), 15 April 1995.

Notes to Chapter 4

70. "Saturday's at Lucy's Beauty Parlor," 20/20 ABC, 13 December 1999. Correspondent Bob Brown.

71. Scott, "Much (2.7 billion) Ado About Hairdos," *Pageant*, May 1962, 124–30, in Peter Tamony Collection, Box 344, under "Hair." On the lives of postwar women see Stephanie Coontz, *The Way We Never Were: American Families and the Nostalgia Trap* (New York: Basic Books, 1992); Joanne Meyerowitz, *Not June Cleaver: Women and Gender in Postwar America, 1945–1960* (Philadelphia: Temple University Press, 1994).

72. The discussion of hairdressers as international celebrities is from *Women's Wear Daily* quoted in Kathrin Perutz, *Beyond the Looking Glass: America's Beauty Culture*, (New York: William Morrow, 1970), 83–84. Also see Jane Howard, Close-Up: George Master's High-Handed Hairdresser," *Life*, 25 November 1966, 57–61, in Peter Tamony Collection, Box 63, under "Beauty Shop."

73. "Airlift May Get In Your Hair, Milady,'" *San Francisco Examiner*, 9 October 1961, 18, in Peter Tamony Collection, Box 345, under "Hair."

74. Scott, "Much (2.7 billion) Ado About Hairdos," *Pageant*, May 1962, 124–30, in Peter Tamony Collection, Box 344, under "Hair."

75. Alice Murray, "Reader Talk: Compassion, Determination and Hardwork," *Shoptalk*, Spring, 1988, 10–12.

76. "For Profit—How She Does It!," *The American Hairdresser*, September 1951, 59.

77. Avis Splies, "Babies Keep Customers Away . . . Here's How Babies Can Bring Them In," *The American Hairdresser*, October 1951, 34.

78. "For Profit—How She Does It!," *The American Hairdresser*, September 1951, 59.

79. *Employment Opportunities for Women in Beauty Service*, 12.

80. Kessler-Harris, *Out to Work*, 302.

81. *Employment Opportunities for Women in Beauty Service*, 6, 12, 30.

82. Cobble, *Dishing It Out*, 118.

83. MAR-106 (1-2), Oral History Collection Chicago Polonia, Chicago Historical Society, Chicago, Illinois, 24–27.

84. "Hazel Foster Proves That 'You Reap What You Sow,'" *Shoptalk*, Fall 1988, 11.

1. Carl Rowan, "Reactions to a Strong Column About African Hair Styles," *San Francisco Examiner*, 12 March 1973, in Peter Tamony Collection, Box 514, under "Afro."

2. Russell Baker, "The Tyranny of a Haircut," *San Francisco Chronicle*, 26 September 1965, in Peter Tamony Collection, Box 344, under "Hair."

3. Bill Severn, *The Long and Short of It* ,1–2, 12.

4. "Would You Cut Your Hair For $50?" *San Francisco Chronicle*, 25 October 1967, in Peter Tamony Collection, Box 344, under "Hair."

5. "Long Hair and Sideburns—The 'In' Look in N.Y." *San Francisco Chronicle*, 28 September 1967, in Peter Tamony Collection, Box 344, under "Hair."

6. Severn, *The Long and Short of It*, 8.

7. Megan Barrett, "Barbershop Boys," *Columbia Missourian*, 12 February 1995.

8. "Would You Use a Beauty Shop for Men?" *San Francisco Chronicle*, 22 August 1967, in Peter Tamony Collection, Box 63, under "Beauty Shop."

9. Interview with Francis Smith, November 1994, Columbia, Missouri.

10. Merla Zellerbach, "Natural Look Or a Disaster?" *San Francisco Chronicle*, 20 November 1972, in Peter Tamony Collection, Box 514, under "Natural Look."

11. "Barbers Boycotting Longhairs' Shops," *San Francisco Chronicle*, 27 January 1971, in Peter Tamony Collection, Box 344, under "Hair."

12. Interview with Leslie Peterson, October 1995, Columbia, Missouri.

13. Robert Mugnai, "How Are The Men In Your Life?" *American Hairdresser Salon Owner*, August 1982, 2.

14. Barrett, "Barber Shop Boys."

15. See Peter Tamony Collection, Box 344, under "Hair," for numerous and varied accounts concerning the "appropriate" length of hair for school children, college students, and employees working in a variety of jobs and locations across the country. For example, see Maitland Zane, "Taxicab Hair Dispute," *San Francisco Chronicle*, 14 April 1970; "Hair 'Hazard' For Fireman," *San Francisco Chronicle*, 21 June 1970; Tom Hall, "Judge Ponders Problem of Long-Haired Athletes,"*San Francisco Examiner*, 21 February 1970; "Longhair

Ban At Disneyland," *San Francisco Chronicle*, 7 August 1970. "David's Back in School After Year of Long Hair," *San Francisco Chronicle*, 18 September 1972.

16. "Fatal Fight Over Son's Hair," *San Francisco Chronicle*, 14 April 1971, in Peter Tamony Collection, Box 344, under "Hair."

17. Ann Landers, "Hassle Over Haircut," *San Francisco Examiner*, 23 April 1968, in Peter Tamony Collection, Box 344, under "Hair"; Ann Landers, "An Exception On Hair," *San Francisco Examiner*, 28 June 1971, in Peter Tamony Collection, Box 344, under "Hair"; Ann Landers, "Jesus' Hair," *San Francisco Examiner*, 5 September 1971, in Peter Tamony Collection, Box 344, under "Hair."

18. Joshua B. Freeman, "Hardhats: Construction Workers, Manliness, and the 1970 Pro-War Demonstrations," *Journal of Social History* 26 (summer 1993): 725–44.

19. First quote from printed letter in Abigail Van Buren, "Hair! Hair! Hair!" *San Francisco Chronicle*, 18 April 1971, in Peter Tamony Collection, Box 344, under "Hair"; second quote from Abigail Van Buren, "The Homemaker vs. the Tired Jobholder," *San Francisco Chronicle*, 31 May 1967, in Peter Tamony Collection, Box 344, under "Hair."

20. "Boy Longhairs Close Up Shop," *San Francisco Examiner*, 13 March 1969, in Peter Tamony Collection, Box 344, under "Hair."

21. Joseph Whitney, "Sons vs. Fathers Over Long Hair," *San Francisco Examiner*, 19 April 1967, in Peter Tamony Collection, Box 344, under "Hair."

22. Chauncey, *Gay New York*, 6–7.

23. David Schroder, *Engagement in the Mirror: Hairdressers and Their Work* (San Francisco: R & E Research Associates, 1978), 23, 59.

24. Bérubé, *Coming Out Under Fire*, 57.

25. Schroder, *Engagement in the Mirror*, 38, 54.

26. "Courting the Male Market," *American Hairdresser Salon Owner*, August, 1982, 60–63.

27. Janet Key, "'Hair Salons' Displace Beauty, Barber Shops," *Chicago Tribune*, 11 February 1985.

28. Beverly Stephen, "Hairdressers—The New Sex Symbol?" *San Francisco Chronicle*, 18 March 1975, in Peter Tamony Collection, Box 345, under "Hairdresser". See also *The New York Times* review by Vincent Canby, "'Shampoo's' Jaundiced Hindsight," reprinted

in the *San Francisco Chronicle*, 23 March 1975, in Peter Tamony Collection, Box 345, under "Hairdresser."

29. Merla Zellerbach, "Beauty in the Barber Shop," *San Francisco Chronicle*, 10 July 1974, in Peter Tamony Collection, Box 63 under "Beauty Shop." See also Merla Zellerbach, "Beauty Shop—Out of Style?" 4 September 1972, in Peter Tamony Collection, Box 63, under "Beauty Shop."

30. David Bouchier, "What Unisex Hair Styling Has Wrought," *New York Times*, 6 November 1994.

31. Key, "'Hair Salons' Displace Beauty, Barber Shops;" Horst Brand and Ziaul Z. Ahmed, "Beauty and Barber Shops: The Trend of Labor Productivity," *Monthly Labor Review*, March 1986, 21–26.

32. Mike Davis, *City of Quartz: Excavating the Future in Los Angeles* (New York: Vintage Books, 1992), 221–64.

33. Interview with Francis Smith.

34. Interview with Janet Thompson, January 1995, Kansas City, Missouri.

35. Interview with Janet Thompson; interview with Leslie Peterson.

36. Interview with Monica Rogers, October 1995, Columbia, Missouri.

37. Interviews with Janet Thompson and Leslie Peterson.

38. Interviews with Leslie Peterson and Francis Smith; interview with Tammy Smith, November 1994, Columbia, Missouri.

39. Interview with Jamie Anderson, May 1995, Columbia, Missouri.

40. Stephanie Pedersen, "Chain Reaction," *Salon News*, December 1994, 22–23.

41. Interviews with Leslie Peterson and Janet Thompson.

42. Interviews with Leslie Peterson and Janet Thompson.

43. Interview with Janet Thompson

44. Interview with Leslie Peterson.

45. Interview with Derrick Williams, November 1995, Columbia, Missouri.

46. *Employment Opportunities for Women in Beauty Service*, U.S. Department of Labor, Women's Bureau, Bulletin no.260 (Washington, 1956), 4; Louise Kapp Howe, *Pink Collar Workers: Inside the World of Women's Work*, (New York: G. P. Putnam's Sons, 1977), 21.

47. Schroder, *Engagement in the Mirror*, 34, 37.

48. Interview with Janet Thompson.

49. Interviews with Janet Thompson, Tammy Smith, and Leslie Peterson.

Notes to Chapter 5

50. Schroder, *Engagement in the Mirror*, 144, 147.

51. Interviews with Janet Thompson, Jamie Anderson, Leslie Peterson, and Derrick Williams.

52. Freeman, "HardHats: Construction Workers, Manliness, and the 1970 Pro-War Demonstrations," 727–44; Montgomery, *Workers' Control in America*, 12–14; Kelley, *Race Rebels*, 2–3.

53. Schroder, *Engagement in the Mirror*, 168.

54. Ibid., 161.

55. "The Changing Image of the Cosmetologist," *Shoptalk*, July 1991, 26–27.

56. Melosh, *"The Physician's Hand."* See especially chapter 1.

57. Interviews with Francis Smith and Tammy Smith.

58. Bebe Moore Campbell, "What Happened to the Afro?," *Ebony*, Vol. 37 (June 1982): 79–84.

59. Assata Shakur, *Assata: An Autobiography* (Chicago: Lawrence Hill Books, 1987), 31, 174–75.

60. Campbell, "What Happened to the Afro?"

61. Dinah Prince, "Who 'Discovered' Cornrows—Bo Derek or Black Women?" *San Francisco Examiner*, 26 March 1980, in Peter Tamony Collection, Box 195, under "Cornrows."

62. Marshall Schwartz, "Doctor's Warning: Afros May Cause Hair Loss," *San Francisco Chronicle*, 22 June 1972, in Peter Tamony Collection, Box 8, under "Afro."

63. "Baldness Peril in Afros, Medic Warns," *San Francisco Examiner*, 22 June 1972, in Peter Tamony, Collection, Box 344, under "Hair"; Marshall Schwartz, "Doctor's Warning: Afros May Cause Hair Loss, *San Francisco Chronicle*, 22 June 1972, in Peter Tamony Collection, Box 8, under "Afro."

64. Don Wegars, "Doctor vs. Stylist: Some Head-Shaking Over Afro Report, *San Francisco Chronicle*, 23 June 1972, in Peter Tamony Collection, Box 8, under "Afro."

65. "Are You Pleased With Your Hairstyle?" *San Francisco Chronicle*, 8 June 1971, in Peter Tamony Collection, Box 8, under "Afro."

66. George Rhodes, "Greyhound Bosses Stomp on Driver's Heels," *San Francisco Examiner*, 4 May 1974, in Peter Tamony Collection, Box 8, under "Afro."

67. Tim Reiterman, "Reporter Stands to Lose Her Job in Hair Dispute," *San Francisco Examiner*, 28 January 1981, in Peter Tamony Collection, Box 195, under "Cornrows"; Harry Jupiter, "Cornrow Case

Settled 'Amicably,'" *San Francisco Chronicle*, 7 February 1981, in Peter Tamony Collection, Box 195, under "Cornrows"; Evelyn Hsu, "Black Reporter's Cornrow Compromise," *San Francisco Chronicle*, 11 February 1981, in Peter Tamony Collection, Box 195, under "Cornrows."

68. Wiley, *Why Black People Tend to Shout*, 8–9, 13.
69. Severn, *The Long and Short of It*, 3.
70. Roediger, *Wages of Whiteness*, 172.
71. Interview with Janet Thompson.
72. Severn, *The Long and Short of It*, 3.
73. Kelley, *Race Rebels*, 2–3, 9.
74. Robert Weems, "The Revolution Will be Marketed: American Corporations and Black Consumers During the 1960s," *Radical History Review*, no. 59 (spring 1994): 94–107. See also Weems, *Desegregating the Dollar*, especially chapter 4.
75. Yla Eason, "Battle of the Beauticians," *Black Enterprise*, November 1980, 32–39; Weems, *Desegregating the Dollar*, 94.
76. Weems, "The Revolution Will be Marketed," 105; Weems, *Desegregating the Dollar*, 70.
77. Yla Eason, "Battle of the Beauticians." See also Robert Mugnai, "The Youth Market! The Ethnic Client! Are You Reaching Them?" *The American Salon*, November 1984, 8,84,26D,28D.
78. Weems, "The Revolution Will be Marketed," 103–4.
79. Eason, "Battle of the Beauticians."
80. Lisa Jones, *Bulletproof Diva: Tales of Race, Sex and Hair* (New York: Doubleday, 1994), 299.
81. Mugnai, "The Youth Market," 8, 24, 26D, 28D.
82. Interview with Francis Smith.
83. Eason, "Battle of the Beauticians."
84. Interviews with Francis Smith and Tammy Smith; Eason, "Battle of the Beautician."
85. Interviews with Monica Rogers and Janet Thompson.
86. Interview with Derrick Williams.
87. Ibid.
88. Interviews with Derrick Williams, Francis Smith, and Tammy Smith
89. Interview with Leslie Peterson.
90. Dennis E. Hensley, "The Advantages of A Small Operation," *Shoptalk*, Spring 1984, 23–32. For a good discussion of the skill

needed to create black hair styles see Lonnice Brittenum Bonner, *Good Hair: For Colored Girls Who've Considered Weaves When the Chemicals Became Too Ruff,* (New York: Crown, 1990). On the intricacy of black hair styles see Bill Gaskins, *Good and Bad Hair* (New Brunswick: Rutgers University Press, 1999).

91. Interview with Derrick Williams.

92. Interviews with Tammy Smith, Monica Rogers, and Leslie Peterson.

93. Interviews with Derrick Williams and Leslie Peterson.

94. Tonia L. Shakespeare, "Hairy Situation, Profitable Business," *Black Enterprise*, April 1995, 31.

95. Jane Applegate, "Cutting Across Cultural Lines," *Los Angeles Times*, 12 December 1988. In my interview with Derrick Williams, his discussion of this topic makes clear that "family salon" meant whiteness in the corporate setting.

96. Patricia Hill Collins, "Learning from the Outsider Within: The Sociological Significance of Black Feminist Thought," *Social Problems* 33, no.6 (December, 1986): 14–32.

97. Interviews with Judith Miller, December 1994, Columbia, Missouri and Derrick Williams.

98. Hensley, "The Advantages of a Small Operation."

99. Applegate, "Cutting Across Cultural Lines."

100. Ibid.

101. Interviews with Judith Miller and Angela Roberts.

102. Interviews with Derrick Williams, Angela Roberts, and Judith Miller.

103. Hensley, "The Advantages of a Small Operation."

104. Loïc J. D. Wacquant, "The New Urban Color Line: The State and Fate of the Ghetto in PostFordist America," in *Social Theory and the Politics of Identity*, ed. Craig Calhoun, (Oxford: Blackwell Publishers, 1994), 238–39; on the collapse of America's manufacturing base see also Howard P. Chudacoff and Judith E. Smith, *The Evolution of American Urban Society*, Third Edition (New Jersey: Prentice Hall, 1988).

105. Interview with Derrick Williams.

106. Interviews with Derrick Williams and Judith Miller.

107. Andy Steiner, "Beauty Shop Docs: In California, Hairdressers Are Also Healers," *UTNE Reader*, January–February 1998, 18.

108. Interview with Derrick Williams.

Notes to Chapter 5

109. Wiley, *Why Black People Tend to Shout*, 11.
110. Hensley, "The Advantages of a Small Salon Operation."

Note to the Conclusion

1. "Bloomie's Discrimination Alleged," *Pioneer Press* (St. Paul, Minn.) 24 August 1996.

Bibliography

Amott, Teresa L., and Julie A. Matthaei. *Race, Gender, and Work: A Multicultural Economic History of Women in the United States*. Boston: South End Press, 1991.

Bailey, Beth. *From Front Porch to Back Seat: Courtship in Twentieth-Century America*. Baltimore: Johns Hopkins University Press, 1988.

Banner, Lois. *American Beauty*. Chicago: University of Chicago Press, 1983.

Berg, Charles. *The Unconscious Significance of Hair*. Leicester: Blackfriars Press, 1951.

Bérubé, Allan. *Coming Out under Fire: The History of Gay Men and Women in World War Two*. New York: Penguin Books, 1991.

Boris, Eileen, and Cynthia R. Daniels, eds., *Homework: Historical and Contemporary Perspectives on Paid Labor at Home*. Urbana: University of Illinois Press, 1989.

Braverman, Harry. *Labor and Monopoly Capital: The Degradation of Work in the Twentieth Century*. New York: Monthly Review Press, 1974.

Breines, Wini. *Young, White, and Miserable: Growing Up Female in the Fifties*. Boston: Beacon Press, 1992.

Brooks Higginbotham, Evelyn. *Righteous Discontent: The Women's Movement in the Black Baptist Church, 1880–1920*. Cambridge: Harvard University Press, 1993.

Brittenum Bonner, Lonnice. *Good Hair: For Colored Girls Who've Considered Weaves When the Chemicals Become Too Ruff*. New York: Crown, 1992.

Cameron, Ardis. *Radicals of the Worst Sort: Laboring Women in Lawrence, Massachusetts, 1860–1912*. Urbana: University of Illinois Press, 1993.

Carnes, Mark. *Secret Ritual and Manhood in Victorian America*. New Haven: Yale University Press, 1989.

Chauncey, George. *Gay New York: Gender, Urban Culture, and the Making of the Gay World, 1890–1940*. New York: Basic Books, 1994.

Chudacoff Howard P., and Smith, Judith E. *The Evolution of American Urban Society*. 3d ed. New Jersey: Prentice Hall, 1988.

Clark Sadler, Georgia. "From Women's Services to Servicewomen." In *Gender Camouflage: Women and the U.S. Military*, ed. Francine D'Amico and Laurie Weinstein, pp. 39–54. New York: New York University Press, 1999.

Clark-Lewis, Elizabeth. *Living In, Living Out: African American Domestics and the Great Migration*. Washington, D.C.: Smithsonian Institution Press, 1984.

———. "'This Work Had a End': African-American Domestic Workers in Washington, D.C., 1910–1940." In *"To Toil the Livelong Day": America's Women at Work, 1780–1980*, ed. Carole Groneman and Mary Beth Norton, pp. 196–212. Ithaca: Cornell University Press, 1987.

Clawson, Mary Ann. *Constructing Brotherhood: Class, Gender, and Fraternalism*. Princeton: Princeton University Press, 1983.

Cobble, Dorothy Sue. *Dishing It Out: Waitresses and Their Unions in the Twentieth Century*. Urbana: University of Illinois Press, 1991.

Cohen, Lizabeth. *Making a New Deal: Industrial Workers in Chicago, 1919–1939*. Cambridge: Cambridge University Press, 1990.

Connolly, Ida. *Beauty Operator on Broadway*. Fresno: Academy Library Guild, 1954.

Coontz, Stephanie. *The Way We Never Were: American Families and the Nostalgia Trap*. New York: Basic Books, 1992.

Cooper, Wendy. *Hair: Sex, Society, Symbolism*. New York: Stein and Day, 1971.

Davis, Mike. *City of Quartz: Excavating the Future in Los Angeles*. New York: Vintage Books, 1992.

Dowd Hall, Jacquelyn. *Like a Family: The Making of a Southern Cotton Mill World*. Chapel Hill: University of North Carolina Press, 1987.

Ewen, Elizabeth. *Immigrant Women in the Land of Dollars: Life and Culture on the Lower East Side, 1890–1925*. New York: Monthly Review Press, 1985.

D'Emilio, John, and Estelle B. Freedman. *Intimate Matters: A History of*   **237**
Sexuality in America. New York: Harper and Row, 1988.

Drake, St. Clair, and Horace R. Cayton. *Black Metropolis: A Study of Negro Life in a Northern City.* 3d rev. ed. New York: Harcourt, Brace and Company, 1945.

Du Bois, W. E. B. *Black Reconstruction in America, 1860–1880.* New York: Atheneum Publishers, 1935.

———. *The Philadelphia Negro: A Social Study.* New York: Noble Offset Printers, 1967.

Dudden, Faye E. *Serving Women: Household Service in Nineteenth-Century America.* Middletown, Conn.: Wesleyan University Press, 1983.

Foff Paules, Greta. *Dishing It Out: Power and Resistance among Waitresses in a New Jersey Restaurant.* Philadelphia: Temple University Press, 1991.

Fox-Genovese, Elizabeth. *Within the Plantation Household: Black and White Women of the Old South.* Chapel Hill: University of North Carolina Press, 1988.

Frank, Miriam, Marilyn Ziebarth, and Connie Field. *The Life and Times of Rosie the Riveter: The Story of Three Million Working Women During World War II.* Emeryville, Calif.: Clarity Educational Productions, 1982.

Freeman, Joshua. "Hardhats: Construction Workers, Manliness, and the 1970 Pro-War Demonstrations." *Journal of Social History* 26 (summer 1993): 725–44.

Gaines, Kevin. *Uplifting the Race: Black Leadership, Politics, and Culture in the Twentieth Century.* Chapel Hill: University of North Carolina Press, 1996.

Gamber, Wendy. *The Female Economy: The Millinery and Dressmaking Trades, 1860–1930.* Urbana: University of Illinois Press, 1997.

Gaskins, Bill. *Good and Bad Hair.* New Brunswick: Rutgers University Press, 1999.

Gilmore, Glenda Elizabeth. *Gender and Jim Crow: Women and the Politics of White Supremacy in North Carolina, 1896–1920.* Chapel Hill: University of North Carolina Press, 1996.

Gray White, Deborah. *Ar'n't I A Woman: Female Slaves in the Plantation South.* New York: Norton, 1985.

Green, Harvey. *Fit for America: Health, Fitness, Sport, and American Society.* Baltimore: John Hopkins University Press, 1986.

238   Grossman, James R. *Land of Hope: Chicago, Black Southerners, and the Great Migration*. Chicago: University of Chicago Press, 1989.

Hareven, Tamara K., and John Modell. "Urbanization and the Malleable Household: An Examination of Boarding and Lodging in American Families." *Journal of Marriage and the Family* 35 (August 1973): 467–79.

Hartman Strom, Sharon. *Beyond the Typewriter: Gender, Class, and the Origins of Modern American Office Work, 1900–1930*. Urbana: University of Illinois Press, 1992.

Hawley, Ellis W. *The New Deal and the Problem of Monopoly: A Study in Economic Ambivalence*. Princeton: Princeton University Press, 1966.

Higham, John. *Strangers in the Land: Patterns of American Nativism*. New Brunswick: Rutgers University Press, 1955.

Hill Collins, Patricia. "Learning from the Outsider Within: The Sociological Significance of Black Feminist Thought." *Social Problems* 33, no.6 (December 1986): 15–32.

hooks, bell. *Ain't I A Woman: Black Women and Feminism*. Boston: South End Press, 1981.

———. *Black Looks: Race and Representation*. Boston: South End Press, 1992.

Hunter, Tera W. *"To 'Joy My Freedom": Southern Black Women's Lives and Labors after the Civil War*. Cambridge: Harvard University Press, 1997.

Jacobs, Harriet. *Incidents in the Life of a Slave Girl*. New York: Oxford University Press, 1988.

Jacobs, Nathan E., ed. *NHCA's Golden Years*. Racine, Wis.: Western, 1970.

Jones, Jacqueline. *Labor of Love, Labor of Sorrow: Black Women, Work, and the Family From Slavery to the Present*. New York: Vintage Books, 1985.

Jones, Lisa. *Bulletproof Diva: Tales of Race, Sex, and Hair*. New York: Doubleday, 1994.

Kapp Howe, Louise. *Pink Collar Workers: Inside the World of Women's Work*. New York: G. P. Putnam's Sons, 1977.

Kelley, Robin D. G. *Race Rebels: Culture, Politics, and the Black Working Class*. New York: Free Press, 1994.

Kerner Furman, Frida. *Facing the Mirror: Older Women and Beauty Shop Culture*. New York: Routledge, 1997.

Kessler-Harris, Alice. *Out to Work: A History of Wage Earning Women in the United States.* New York: Oxford University Press, 1982.

Kessner, Thomas. *The Golden Door: Italian and Jewish Immigrant Mobility in New York, 1880–1915.* New York: Oxford University Press, 1977.

Kingsdale, Jon. "The 'Poor Man's Club': Social Functions of the Urban Working-Class Saloon." In *The American Man*, ed. Elizabeth Pleck and Joseph Pleck, pp. 255–83. Englewood Cliffs, N.J.: Prentice Hall, 1980.

Knobel, Dale T. *America for the Americans: The Nativist Movement in the United States.* New York: Twayne Publishers, 1996.

Kuhn, Clifford M., Harlon E. Joye, and E. Bernard West. *Living Atlanta: An Oral History of the City, 1914–1948.* Athens: University of Georgia Press, 1990.

Lott, Eric. *Love and Theft: Blackface Minstrelsy and the American Working Class.* New York: Oxford University Press, 1993.

Marable, Manning. *How Capitalism Underdeveloped Black America: Problems in Race, Political Economy, and Society.* Boston: South End Press, 1983.

———. *Race, Reform, and Rebellion: The Second Reconstruction in Black America, 1945–1990.* Jackson: University Press of Mississippi, 1991.

McAdam, Doug. *Political Process and the Development of Black Insurgency 1930–1970.* Chicago: University of Chicago Press, 1982.

McBee, Randy D. *Dance Hall Days: Intimacy and Leisure among Working-Class Immigrants in the United States.* New York: New York University Press, forthcoming.

Melosh, Barbara. *"The Physician's Hand": Work Culture and Conflict in American Nursing.* Philadelphia: Temple University Press, 1982.

Mercer, Kobena. "Black Hair/Black Style." In *Out There: Marginalization and Contemporary Cultures*, ed. Russell Ferguson et al., pp. 247–64. Cambridge: Massachusetts Institute for Technology Press, 1990.

Meyerowitz, Joanne. *Not June Cleaver: Women and Gender in Postwar America, 1945–1960.* Philadelphia: Temple University Press, 1994.

Milkman, Ruth. *Gender at Work: The Dynamics of Job Segregation by Sex during World War II.* Urbana: University of Illinois Press, 1987.

Montgomery, David. *Workers' Control in America: Studies in the History of Work, Technology, and Labor Struggles.* Cambridge: Cambridge University Press, 1979.

Moody, Anne. *Coming of Age in Mississippi.* New York: Dell, 1968.

Morris, Aldon. *The Origins of the Civil Rights Movement: Black Communities Organizing for Change.* New York: Free Press, 1984.

Mumford, Kevin J. *Interzones: Black/White Sex Districts in Chicago and New York in the Early Twentieth Century.* New York: Columbia University Press, 1997.

Nasaw, David. *Going Out: The Rise and Fall of Public Amusements.* New York: Basic Books, 1993.

Neth, Mary. *Preserving the Family Farm: Women, Community, and the Foundations of Agribusiness in the Midwest, 1900–1940.* Baltimore: Johns Hopkins University Press, 1995.

Orsi, Robert. "The Religious Boundaries of an Inbetween People: Street Feste and the Problem of the Dark-Skinned 'Other' in Italian Harlem, 1920–1990." *American Quarterly* 44 (Sept. 1992): 313–47.

Palmer, Phyllis. *Domesticity and Dirt: Housewives and Domestic Servants in the United States, 1920–1945.* Philadelphia: Temple University Press, 1989.

Patterson, Orlando. *Slavery and Social Death: A Comparative Study.* Cambridge: Harvard University Press, 1982.

Peiss, Kathy. *Cheap Amusements: Working Women and Leisure in Turn-of-the-Century New York.* Philadelphia: Temple University Press, 1986.

———. "Making Faces: The Cosmetics Industry and the Cultural Construction of Gender, 1890–1930." *Genders* 7 (spring 1990): 143–69.

———. *Hope in a Jar: The Making of America's Beauty Culture.* New York: Metropolitan Books, 1998.

Perry Bundles, A'Lelia. *Madam C. J. Walker.* New York: Chelsea House, 1991.

Perutz, Kathrin. *Beyond the Looking Glass: America's Beauty Culture.* New York: William Morrow, 1970.

Porter Benson, Susan. *Counter Cultures: Saleswomen, Managers, and Customers in American Department Stores, 1890–1940.* Urbana: University of Illinois Press, 1986.

Porter, Gladys L. *Three Negro Pioneers in Beauty Culture.* New York: Vantage Press, 1966.

Potter, Eliza. *A Hairdresser's Experience in High Life.* New York: Oxford University Press, 1991.

Bibliography

240

Moody, Anne. *Coming of Age in Mississippi*. New York: Dell, 1968.

Morris, Aldon. *The Origins of the Civil Rights Movement: Black Communities Organizing for Change*. New York: Free Press, 1984.

Mumford, Kevin J. *Interzones: Black/White Sex Districts in Chicago and New York in the Early Twentieth Century*. New York: Columbia University Press, 1997.

Nasaw, David. *Going Out: The Rise and Fall of Public Amusements*. New York: Basic Books, 1993.

Neth, Mary. *Preserving the Family Farm: Women, Community, and the Foundations of Agribusiness in the Midwest, 1900–1940*. Baltimore: Johns Hopkins University Press, 1995.

Orsi, Robert. "The Religious Boundaries of an Inbetween People: Street Feste and the Problem of the Dark-Skinned 'Other' in Italian Harlem, 1920–1990." *American Quarterly* 44 (Sept. 1992): 313–47.

Palmer, Phyllis. *Domesticity and Dirt: Housewives and Domestic Servants in the United States, 1920–1945*. Philadelphia: Temple University Press, 1989.

Patterson, Orlando. *Slavery and Social Death: A Comparative Study*. Cambridge: Harvard University Press, 1982.

Peiss, Kathy. *Cheap Amusements: Working Women and Leisure in Turn-of-the-Century New York*. Philadelphia: Temple University Press, 1986.

———. "Making Faces: The Cosmetics Industry and the Cultural Construction of Gender, 1890–1930." *Genders* 7 (spring 1990): 143–69.

———. *Hope in a Jar: The Making of America's Beauty Culture*. New York: Metropolitan Books, 1998.

Perry Bundles, A'Lelia. *Madam C. J. Walker*. New York: Chelsea House, 1991.

Perutz, Kathrin. *Beyond the Looking Glass: America's Beauty Culture*. New York: William Morrow, 1970.

Porter Benson, Susan. *Counter Cultures: Saleswomen, Managers, and Customers in American Department Stores, 1890–1940*. Urbana: University of Illinois Press, 1986.

Porter, Gladys L. *Three Negro Pioneers in Beauty Culture*. New York: Vantage Press, 1966.

Potter, Eliza. *A Hairdresser's Experience in High Life*. New York: Oxford University Press, 1991.

237

D'Emilio, John, and Estelle B. Freedman. *Intimate Matters: A History of Sexuality in America*. New York: Harper and Row, 1988.

Drake, St. Clair, and Horace R. Cayton. *Black Metropolis: A Study of Negro Life in a Northern City*. 3d rev. ed. New York: Harcourt, Brace and Company, 1945.

Du Bois, W. E. B. *Black Reconstruction in America, 1860–1880*. New York: Atheneum Publishers, 1935.

———. *The Philadelphia Negro: A Social Study*. New York: Noble Offset Printers, 1967.

Dudden, Faye E. *Serving Women: Household Service in Nineteenth-Century America*. Middletown, Conn.: Wesleyan University Press, 1983.

Foff Paules, Greta. *Dishing It Out: Power and Resistance among Waitresses in a New Jersey Restaurant*. Philadelphia: Temple University Press, 1991.

Fox-Genovese, Elizabeth. *Within the Plantation Household: Black and White Women of the Old South*. Chapel Hill: University of North Carolina Press, 1988.

Frank, Miriam, Marilyn Ziebarth, and Connie Field. *The Life and Times of Rosie the Riveter: The Story of Three Million Working Women During World War II*. Emeryville, Calif.: Clarity Educational Productions, 1982.

Freeman, Joshua. "Hardhats: Construction Workers, Manliness, and the 1970 Pro-War Demonstrations." *Journal of Social History* 26 (summer 1993): 725–44.

Gaines, Kevin. *Uplifting the Race: Black Leadership, Politics, and Culture in the Twentieth Century*. Chapel Hill: University of North Carolina Press, 1996.

Gamber, Wendy. *The Female Economy: The Millinery and Dressmaking Trades, 1860–1930*. Urbana: University of Illinois Press, 1997.

Gaskins, Bill. *Good and Bad Hair*. New Brunswick: Rutgers University Press, 1999.

Gilmore, Glenda Elizabeth. *Gender and Jim Crow: Women and the Politics of White Supremacy in North Carolina, 1896–1920*. Chapel Hill: University of North Carolina Press, 1996.

Gray White, Deborah. *Ar'n't I A Woman: Female Slaves in the Plantation South*. New York: Norton, 1985.

Green, Harvey. *Fit for America: Health, Fitness, Sport, and American Society*. Baltimore: John Hopkins University Press, 1986.

238 Grossman, James R. *Land of Hope: Chicago, Black Southerners, and the Great Migration.* Chicago: University of Chicago Press, 1989.

Hareven, Tamara K., and John Modell. "Urbanization and the Malleable Household: An Examination of Boarding and Lodging in American Families." *Journal of Marriage and the Family* 35 (August 1973): 467–79.

Hartman Strom, Sharon. *Beyond the Typewriter: Gender, Class, and the Origins of Modern American Office Work, 1900–1930.* Urbana: University of Illinois Press, 1992.

Hawley, Ellis W. *The New Deal and the Problem of Monopoly: A Study in Economic Ambivalence.* Princeton: Princeton University Press, 1966.

Higham, John. *Strangers in the Land: Patterns of American Nativism.* New Brunswick: Rutgers University Press, 1955.

Hill Collins, Patricia. "Learning from the Outsider Within: The Sociological Significance of Black Feminist Thought." *Social Problems* 33, no.6 (December 1986): 15–32.

hooks, bell. *Ain't I A Woman: Black Women and Feminism.* Boston: South End Press, 1981.

———. *Black Looks: Race and Representation.* Boston: South End Press, 1992.

Hunter, Tera W. *"To 'Joy My Freedom": Southern Black Women's Lives and Labors after the Civil War.* Cambridge: Harvard University Press, 1997.

Jacobs, Harriet. *Incidents in the Life of a Slave Girl.* New York: Oxford University Press, 1988.

Jacobs, Nathan E., ed. *NHCA's Golden Years.* Racine, Wis.: Western, 1970.

Jones, Jacqueline. *Labor of Love, Labor of Sorrow: Black Women, Work, and the Family From Slavery to the Present.* New York: Vintage Books, 1985.

Jones, Lisa. *Bulletproof Diva: Tales of Race, Sex, and Hair.* New York: Doubleday,1994.

Kapp Howe, Louise. *Pink Collar Workers: Inside the World of Women's Work.* New York: G. P. Putnam's Sons, 1977.

Kelley, Robin D. G. *Race Rebels: Culture, Politics, and the Black Working Class.* New York: Free Press, 1994.

Kerner Furman, Frida. *Facing the Mirror: Older Women and Beauty Shop Culture.* New York: Routledge, 1997.

Kessler-Harris, Alice. *Out to Work: A History of Wage Earning Women in the United States.* New York: Oxford University Press, 1982.

Kessner, Thomas. *The Golden Door: Italian and Jewish Immigrant Mobility in New York, 1880–1915.* New York: Oxford University Press, 1977.

Kingsdale, Jon. "The 'Poor Man's Club': Social Functions of the Urban Working-Class Saloon." In *The American Man,* ed. Elizabeth Pleck and Joseph Pleck, pp. 255–83. Englewood Cliffs, N.J.: Prentice Hall, 1980.

Knobel, Dale T. *America for the Americans: The Nativist Movement in the United States.* New York: Twayne Publishers, 1996.

Kuhn, Clifford M., Harlon E. Joye, and E. Bernard West. *Living Atlanta: An Oral History of the City, 1914–1948.* Athens: University of Georgia Press, 1990.

Lott, Eric. *Love and Theft: Blackface Minstrelsy and the American Working Class.* New York: Oxford University Press, 1993.

Marable, Manning. *How Capitalism Underdeveloped Black America: Problems in Race, Political Economy, and Society.* Boston: South End Press, 1983.

———. *Race, Reform, and Rebellion: The Second Reconstruction in Black America, 1945–1990.* Jackson: University Press of Mississippi, 1991.

McAdam, Doug. *Political Process and the Development of Black Insurgency 1930–1970.* Chicago: University of Chicago Press, 1982.

McBee, Randy D. *Dance Hall Days: Intimacy and Leisure among Working-Class Immigrants in the United States.* New York: New York University Press, forthcoming.

Melosh, Barbara. *"The Physician's Hand": Work Culture and Conflict in American Nursing.* Philadelphia: Temple University Press, 1982.

Mercer, Kobena. "Black Hair/Black Style." In *Out There: Marginalization and Contemporary Cultures,* ed. Russell Ferguson et al., pp. 247–64. Cambridge: Massachusetts Institute for Technology Press, 1990.

Meyerowitz, Joanne. *Not June Cleaver: Women and Gender in Postwar America, 1945–1960.* Philadelphia: Temple University Press, 1994.

Milkman, Ruth. *Gender at Work: The Dynamics of Job Segregation by Sex during World War II.* Urbana: University of Illinois Press, 1987.

Montgomery, David. *Workers' Control in America: Studies in the History of Work, Technology, and Labor Struggles.* Cambridge: Cambridge University Press, 1979.

Rawick, George. *From Sundown to Sunup: The Making of the Black Community*. Westport, Conn.: Greenwood Press, 1972.

Rediker, Marcus. *Between the Devil and the Deep Blue Sea: Merchant Seamen, Pirates, and the Anglo-American Maritime World, 1700–1750*. Cambridge: Cambridge University Press, 1987.

Robinson, Gwendolyn. "Class, Race and Gender: A Transcultural, Theoretical and Sociohistorical Analysis of Cosmetic Institutions and Practices to 1920." Ph.D. diss., University of Illinois at Chicago, 1984.

Roediger, David. *Wages of Whiteness: Race and the Making of the American Working Class*. London: Verso, 1991.

Rooks, Noliwe. *Hair Rasing: Beauty, Culture, and African American Women*. New Brunswick: Rutgers University Press, 1996.

Rosenzweig, Roy. *Eight Hours for What We Will: Workers and Leisure in an Industrial City, 1870–1920*. Cambridge: Cambridge University Press, 1983.

Ruiz, Vicki L. "The Flapper and the Chaperone: Historical Memory among Mexican-American Women." In *Seeking Common Ground: Multidisciplinary Studies of Immigrant Women in the United States*, ed. Donna Gabaccia, pp. 141–58. Westport, Conn.: Greenwood Press, 1992.

Russell Hochschild, Arlie. *The Managed Heart: Commercialization of Human Feeling*. Berkeley: University of California Press, 1983.

Sagay, Esi. *African Hairstyles: Styles of Yesterday and Today*. London: Heinemann, 1983.

Schroder, David. *Engagement in the Mirror: Hairdressers and Their Work*. San Francisco: R & E Research Associates, 1978.

Severn, Bill. *The Long and Short of It: Five Thousand Years of Fun and Fury over Hair*. New York: David McKay, 1971.

Shakur, Assata. *Assata: An Autobiography*. Chicago: Lawrence Hill Books, 1987.

Shapiro, Herbert. *White Violence and Black Response: From Reconstruction to Montgomery*. Amherst: University of Massachusetts Press, 1988.

Simmons, Christina. "Companionate Marriage and the Lesbian Threat." *Frontiers* 4, no. 3 (1979): 54–59.

———. "Modern Sexuality and the Myth of Victorian Repression." In *Passion and Power: Sexuality in History*, ed. Kathy Peiss and Christina Simmons, pp. 157–77. Philadelphia: Temple University Press, 1989.

242   Smith-Rosenberg, Carroll. "Discourses of Sexuality and Subjectivity: The New Woman 1870–1936." In *Hidden From History: Reclaiming the Gay and Lesbian Past*, ed. Martin Dubermann et al., pp. 264–80. New York: Meridian, 1990.

Spear, Alan H. *Black Chicago: The Making of a Negro Ghetto, 1890–1920*. Chicago: University of Chicago Press, 1967.

Stahl Weinberg, Sydney. *The World of Our Mothers: The Lives of Jewish Immigrant Women*. Chapel Hill: University of North Carolina Press, 1988.

Stuckey, Sterling. *Going through The Storm: The Influence of African American Art in History*. New York: Oxford University Press, 1994.

Thompson, E. P. *The Making of the English Working Class*. New York: Vintage, 1966.

Trotter, Joe William. *Black Milwaukee: The Making of an Industrial Proletariat, 1915–1945*. Urbana: University of Illinois Press, 1985.

Tyler May, Elaine. *Homeward Bound: American Families in the Cold War Era*. New York: Basic Books, 1988.

Wacquant, Loïc J. D. "The New Urban Line: The State and the Fate of the Ghetto in PostFordist America." In *Social Theory and the Politics of Identity*, ed. Craig Calhoun, pp. 238–39. Oxford: Blackwell Publishers, 1994.

Ware, Susan. *Holding Their Own: American Women in the 1930s*. Boston: Twayne Publishers, 1982.

Weems, Robert. "The Revolution Will Be Marketed: American Corporations and Black Consumers During the 1960s." *Radical History Review* 59 (spring 1994): 94–107.

————. *Desegregating the Dollar: African American Consumerism in the Twentieth Century*. New York: New York University Press, 1998.

White, Shane, and Graham White. *Stylin': African American Expressive Culture from Its Beginnings to the Zoot Suit*. Ithica: Cornell University Press, 1998.

Wigginton, Eliot. *Refuse to Stand Silently By: An Oral History of Grass Roots Social Activism in America, 1921–1964*. New York: Doubleday Dell, 1991.

Wiley, Ralph. *Why Black People Tend to Shout: Cold Facts and Wry Views from a Black Man's World*. New York: Carol, 1991.

Woodward, C. Vann. *The Strange Career of Jim Crow*. 3d rev. ed. Oxford: Oxford University Press, 1974.

Bibliography

Yans-McLaughlin, Virginia. *Family and Community: Italian Immigrants*
in Buffalo, 1880–1930. Urbana: University of Illinois Press, 1982.

Yung, Judy. *Unbound Feet: A Social History of Chinese Women in San Francisco.* Berkeley: University of California Press, 1995.

Index

African-American women: beauty schools, 62; consumption, 19; domestic service, 21–22; health hazards, 94; NRA, 105; politics of respectability, 22; prices, 103; professionalism, 115; wages, 105; white-collar work, 21. *See also* Beauty shop (African American)

Afro, 154, 178; commodification of, 177; controversy surrounding, 179–180; symbol of black pride, 176–177, 178; white reactions to, 180

American Cosmeticians Association, and professionalism, 114–115

American Hairdresser, The: gossip, 82–83; licensing during WWII, 124; model shop, 147–148; patriotic campaigns during WWII, 126; professionalism, 112–114; rural shops, 103; teen market, 136–137; time and motion studies, 142–143; "trouble corner," 72

Anti-permanents, 180. *See also* Afro; Cornrows; Hair straightening

Apprenticeship, 59–60

Banner, Lois, 56

Barber shops, 1, 3; competition from beauty shops, 80; decline of, 157–158; and immigrants, 44–45; and Jim Crow, 44; male culture, 42–43, 156; and prostitution, 45–46; unionization, 80–81; and women, 43–44

Beauty schools: advertisements, 54–55; alternatives to, 57; apprenticeship, 59–60; class distinctions, 57; compared to medical care, 56; competition for students, 58–59; concerns over poorly trained operators, 91; courses, 55, 56; Depression, 111–112; enrollment after WWII, 142; exploitation of students, 112; professionalism, 54–55, 56; racial segregation, 62; regional differences, 57; requirements, 61; training, 55, 56; tuition, 52; unfit workers, 57–58; working-class customers, 59

Beauty shops: air conditioning, 76–77; and barber shops, distinguished from, 118; bartering, 69–70; bathroom shops, 91, 99; before segregation, 18; black customers and white stylists, 186; business practices, 34; classification, 117–119; as community institution, 1–3; as cornerstone of industry, 91; customers and problems, 70–71; decline of, 162; department stores, 98; descriptions of, 63–64, 66–68; equipment and safety, 94, 96; European origins, 30–31; expansion of, 122; expansion, post-WWII, 135–138; factory, during WWII, 127–128; and girlhood, 36; hair care practices before, 26–27; hours of operation, 97–98; inventions by female hairdressers, 32–33; kitchen shops undercutting prices, 99; labor shortage, post-WWII, 140–142; and Latina operators, 194; mishaps, 92–97; moral economy, 102–103; and NRA, support for, 101;

245

About the Author

Julie A. Willett is Assistant Professor of History at Texas Tech University.